How to Do Your Hair Like a Pro

BY
VINCENT AND FRED NARDI
WITH
MARINA MAHER

A GD/PERIGEE BOOK

We wish to thank all our staff who participated in teaching the New School classes—especially Sal, Michael, Sergio, Paul, Lucille, and Franklin.

Deepest love and appreciation to our parents who made our achievements possible.

Perigee Books
are published by
The Putnam Publishing Group
200 Madison Avenue
New York, New York 10016

Library of Congress catalog card number: 77-73926
ISBN 0-399-50821-X

Designed by Marcia Ben-Eli
Illustrations by Ray Skibinski
Cover photographed by Kenn Mori
Cover makeup by Sara McC. Bandy

First Perigee printing, 1983
Four previous Grosset & Dunlap printings
Printed in the United States of America
    2   3   4   5   6   7   8   9

Contents

I'm not right, and I want to learn what to do about it."

Our New School courses were highly successful. Phone calls and letters poured in, asking if we could possibly give this course in other areas. We realized then that there must be people everywhere who need and want help with their hair—people who couldn't go to a class for one reason or another. In this book, we have expanded on the subject matter we taught at the New School, providing information in greater detail. We've also incorporated many questions asked by our students, assuming that your questions might be similar. And we've thoroughly illustrated our instructions, so that our readers can follow step by step, as though they were in our classroom.

This book is for everyone, and for all aspects of hair care. If you've already been doing your own hair, it will give you the know-how to achieve professional-looking results. If you have a family, you'll appreciate the economy of learning how to cut your child's hair or trim Dad's. If you travel frequently, or keep a very busy schedule, you'll learn the secrets of hair maintenance under time pressures. If you're letting your hair grow out, you can learn how to give yourself trims.

For those who go to the hairdresser on a regular basis, it's important to learn a little about the language of hair, to learn what's right and what's wrong for your hair type. Don't go to a stylist and bury your head in a magazine. Watch what's being done and construct your own rating system from what you've learned here.

Anyone's hair can be improved. Whether you want to do it all yourself, or only partly, you'll find the help you need here. So enjoy, experiment, and go to it!

Introduction

The best hairstyle in the world means nothing if you can't handle it on your own!

The era is past—or at least it should be—when women were totally dependent on their hairdressers. At one time women were tied to a standing weekly appointment during which they sat voiceless in the chair while the hairdresser decided what was to be done.

With today's freedom, hair is wash-and-wear, and women take an active part in determining their hairstyles. More important, most women want to know how to maintain their hair. In our salons we have always felt that a client should express her feelings about how her hair is to be cut. And, once that's established, we make sure she understands how to keep up that look—how to style it, how often to wash it, etc.

Since we've always liked teaching our clients about their hair, it was only natural that eventually we should teach an entire course on the subject. And so we taught a class at the New School for Social Research, a New York City college that offers a wide variety of contemporary courses. We called the course "Be Your Own Topnotch Hairdresser," and to the best of our knowledge, it was the only class of its kind ever given.

The course met with immediate success. Women—and men, too—had dozens of questions about how to deal with their hair. And we were delighted to observe that all types of people sought this knowledge. For example, one of our students was a salesman who realized the importance of a good appearance in his job. But, he confided in us, his friends had kidded him about signing up for a class on hair care. After a few classes the salesman's hair had improved greatly, and he was quite happy. Now, he told us, his friends had changed their tune. His phone rang frequently after each class—his friends were calling to find out what he had learned!

Another student was a dancer in a nightclub; she wanted to learn how to make her hair more dramatic for the stage. We even had a nun on our waiting list; she said she wanted "a very different kind of look."

In our classes we taught housewives and career women, teenagers and senior citizens. No matter the age or occupation or sex, they all had one common goal: to learn how to manage their own hair. As we heard repeatedly: "If my hair isn't right,

This book is dedicated to everyone
who wants more beautiful, healthy-looking hair.

1.

How to Determine the Cut and Style Best for You

Choosing the right cut and style is easy, once you understand what works best for you.

In our salons a great deal of thought goes into deciding how to cut a client's hair. First, we discuss with the client what she wants from her hair. Is she more concerned with style or with ease of care, for instance? Then we consider several factors, such as hair type, face shape, and suitability. Only after we have all this information do we suggest several different haircuts.

You should follow much the same routine before cutting your hair at home. This chapter will show you how to go about it. You will analyze your hair type, then we will suggest certain styles that are most compatible with what nature gave you. By analyzing your face shape and feature flaws, you will learn how the right style can enhance your looks. Finally, we will ask questions about your life style so that you can decide how much time you can spend on your hair and how your hair

Haircuts For Your Hair Type

FORMATION	FINE Hair often thin, separates easily

STRAIGHT
(no natural
movement)
	Layered; short
	
	Combination cut: blunt back for
	  body, layered front for
	  movement.
	
	Length: chin to midneck
	
	(See pages 19, 22, 35, 44, 51, 57, 73)

SLIGHTLY WAVY (slight wave pattern)	Layered: short Blunt cut: chin to collarbone Combination cut: blunt back for body, layered front for movement Length: chin to collarbone. *(See pages 19, 22, 25, 29, 35, 41, 44, 51, 57, 67, 73)*
WAVY (definite wave pattern)	Layered: 1½-5 inches Blunt cut: chin length Combination cut: blunt back for body, layered front for movement Length: chin to collarbone *(See pages 19, 22, 29, 35, 41, 44, 51, 57, 67)*
CURLY (falls into cork- screws naturally)	Layered: 3 inches Combination cut: blunt back and sides, slight layers in front Length: chin to collarbone *(See pages 19, 22, 29, 41, 44, 51, 67)*
FRIZZY (tight curls)	Layered: 2½-5 inches Blunt cut: collarbone length *(See pages 19, 22, 41, 44, 51, 57, 67)*

MEDIUM Average amount of hair on head	THICK Full head of hair, sometimes coarse
Blunt cut: chin to shoulder Combination cut: blunt back for body, layered front for movement Length: chin to collarbone *(See pages 19, 22, 25, 29, 35, 44, 51, 57, 73)*	Blunt cut: chin to shoulder (longer gives more control) Combination cut: blunt back for body, layered front for movement Length: chin to collarbone *(See pages 19, 22, 25, 29, 35, 51, 57)*
Layered: short (will show few waves) Blunt cut: chin to collarbone Combination cut: blunt back for body, layered front for movement Length: chin to shoulder *(See pages 19, 22, 25, 29, 35, 41, 44, 51, 57, 67, 73)*	Blunt cut: chin to mid-neck (if longer hair looks bulky) Combination cut: blunt back for body, layered front for movement Length: chin to shoulder *(See pages 19, 22, 29, 35, 41, 51, 67, 73)*
Layered: 3 inches (waves may go into a slight curl) Blunt cut: chin to shoulder Combination cut: blunt back for body, layered front for movement Length: chin to collarbone *(See pages 19, 22, 29, 35, 41, 51, 57, 67)*	Layered: 2 inches Blunt cut: chin to collarbone Combination cut: blunt back for body, layered front for movement Length: chin to shoulder *(See pages 19, 29, 35, 41, 51, 57, 67)*
Layered: 2-4 inches Blunt cut: with angled sides Length: chin to shoulder *(See pages 19, 22, 29, 41, 44, 51, 67)*	Layered: 2-3 inches **Blunt cut:** with angled sides Length: chin to shoulder *(See pages 19, 29, 41, 44, 51, 67)*
Layered: 2-6 inches Blunt cut: collarbone length *(See pages 19, 22, 29, 41, 44, 51, 57, 67)*	Layered: 2-4 inches Blunt cut: collarbone length *(See pages 19, 22, 29, 41, 51, 67)*

must look in the life you lead.

But keep in mind, no rule applies to everyone all the time. For example, if you have fine hair and a small, round face, we might suggest a soft style with wispy bangs. But if you also wear glasses, you might consider eliminating the bangs to show more of your face.

You may wish to try a look that appeals to you but contradicts several of our guidelines. If you like a particular hairstyle, by all means try it, but also try to make some modifications to fit your needs.

Know Your Hair Type

When a client comes into our salon for a haircut, the first thing we study is her hair type. By analyzing the texture of her hair, its thickness, and the way it moves, we can determine a style that is natural for her. Immediately, we eliminate styles that would force her hair to do something that it would not do on its own.

What do you know about the "raw material" you are working with? For example, if you have fine hair, it will not look its best when it is too long. Similarly, tight, curly hair cannot be cut to fall into a smooth, soft pageboy. If you do not know your hair type, you may be trying to make your hair do something it cannot. If so, you will never be satisfied with the results. What's more, your hair will always look contrived rather than natural.

Among the hundreds of clients who have come to our salons, it is rare to meet a woman who is happy with her hair type! One woman's hair is too fine, another's is too thick. One complains of the frizzies, while in the next chair, someone else is bemoaning her superstraight hair. Sound familiar?

We feel we have accomplished something important when our clients and students come to understand and accept their hair type—and then learn to work with it. And this is what we hope to teach you. For, once you understand your hair, you will always be happy with it because you will know exactly what it *can* do.

Two factors determine the kind of hair you have: formation and texture. *Formation* indicates the way the hair shaft bends: is it tightly curled, slightly wavy, or just straight with no bend at all? *Texture* refers to the quality and quantity of your hair: is it fine and thin, or coarse and thick?

We have prepared a chart to help you find the haircuts that are best for your hair type. The headings contain brief descriptions to make finding your type easier. But before you even look at the chart, here is a quick way to help you determine your hair type.

Does your hair have trouble holding a barrette, and is it fairly smooth and silky? Then you obviously have fine hair. When you run a brush through your hair, does it feel as if you're drawing the brush through something substantial? Can you grasp your hair into a fair-sized ponytail? Then your hair runs medium to thick.

In the chart, under the suggestions for hairstyles, you will find page numbers. These are keyed to the cuts in Chapter 2, which you can either copy or use as guidelines for your own creations.

Know Your Face Shape

A second important factor that determines the best haircut for you is the shape of your face.

Analyzing your face's shape takes a very critical and objective eye, something that not everyone has. So why not trust the most honest eye of all—the camera. Study a few recent photos of yourself, and you will soon determine exactly what shape face you have.

All facial shapes fall into six classic categories. Chart 2 lists the basic principles to follow when choosing a hairstyle for your facial shape as well as tips on what hairstyles to avoid.

We devised another trick for our students, which you may want to follow. Slick back all your hair either by wetting or clipping it. Stand in front of your bathroom mirror, under a bright light. Now take a piece of soap and draw the outline of your face in the mirror. Step back, and there you have it—the shape of your face as it really is.

Chart 2. Face Shapes

Type of Face   Round

Description and Recommendations

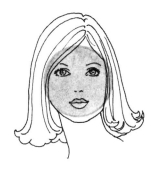

Characteristics: full cheeks, short forehead, no definite chin line

What you need: asymmetrical style, narrowing lines, to expose high point of forehead

What to avoid: straight bangs, any boxy style, roundness in the hairline

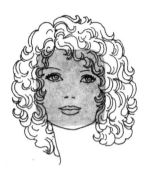

Type of Face Square

Description and Recommendations

Characteristics: strong jawline, wide forehead

What you need: asymmetrical style, softness on top, enough length in back to balance out square line of chin

What to avoid: short hair, very straight lines, too much hair on the face

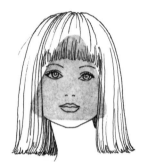

Type of Face Triangle

Description and Recommendations

Characteristics: broad jawline narrowing to forehead

What you need: some width and softness on top; low, wide bangs to camouflage high point of forehead

What to avoid: center parts, anything that falls on the cheekbones

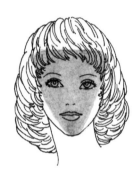

Type of Face Inverted Triangle (Heart-shaped)

Description and Recommendations

Characteristics: broad forehead, tapered jaw, even a pointy chin

What you need: short or long layers on top, side part

What to avoid: bangs, very short cuts, anything severe on top

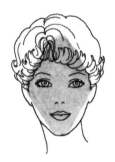

Type of Face Diamond

Description and Recommendations

Characteristics: wide cheekbones, narrow forehead and chin

What you need: soft layers on top, hair brought down softly to center of forehead to camouflage high point of forehead

What to avoid: all hair pulled back, center part

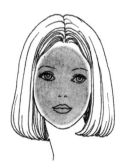

Type of Face Oval

Description and Recommendations

Having an oval face is like being born Sunday's child—you are blessed; wear any style you fancy.

Know Your Features

The right hairstyle can soften a prominent nose or make a jutting jaw recede. It pays to take a good look at your features before deciding on a new hairstyle.

Go back to the mirror and study your features, especially in profile. And be critical; very few features are sculpture-perfect. Is your nose especially noticeable? Does your chin seem to recede? Here are a few tips on what your hairstyle can do about it.

Prominent nose: Straight, hard bangs are not for you. Make sure you have some height and softness at the crown and front. Add some width to the sides. If at times you wear your hair pulled back, make sure it's tied low on the neck so that in profile it doesn't match up with the longest part of your nose.

Short forehead: Expose your forehead so that your face has more length. You can wear bangs if they are soft and slightly see-through, showing the high point of your forehead. Lift side hair up to crown to slenderize forehead.

Long forehead: Wear wide bangs to camouflage a long brow. Add width on the sides, but keep top fairly smooth and low.

Jutting jaw: Since you want to counteract a flaw in the lower portion of your face, concentrate on the top. Make sure there's softness and height on the top. Bring some wisps of hair down on the forehead. Don't wear hair pulled back.

Receding chin: Wear medium-length hairstyles that expose the face or a short cut that lifts hair off the neck. Make sure there's softness throughout crown and front. Pull side hair up toward crown.

Long neck: Wear hair to the shoulder or at least not shorter than mid-neck. Hairstyle should have some volume.

Short neck: To achieve length, expose neck with angle cut.

Know Your Body Shape

Very few people realize the importance of body shape in selecting a hairstyle. But the right hairstyle can be quite effective in offsetting figure problems.

You probably have a good idea of your body shape, but again, it is important to be objective. Don't say, "Well, I'm full-figured now, but I plan to lose fifteen pounds starting next week." Change your hair when you change your weight—not before.

Right now, what is your most basic figure characteristic? Are you short (5'3" and under) or tall (5'7" and over)? Are you on the heavy side or the thin side?

If you're short: Many short women make the mistake of wearing their hair too long, which only makes them look shorter. Wear your hair chin-length or shorter. The style should be soft, not full. If you're thin, you can wear your hair quite short if you like.

If you're tall: Don't wear your hair very close-cropped (especially if you have a long neck), or you will look like a pinhead. Your hair should fall between your chin and your collarbone; make sure that it has some body and fullness.

If you're heavy: Full-figured people should wear neat, fairly simple hairstyles. Anything fussy calls attention to the heaviness. You might want to add interest with hair coloring. Choose a shade that highlights your natural hair color. Length can be anywhere from chin to collarbone.

If you're thin: Thin people have fewer limitations than most, but they should stay away from styles with an abundance of hair; this is generally overpowering to the person with a thin figure. If you want long hair, make sure your face is exposed.

What's Your Life Style?

You have thought about your hair and about how it relates to your face and body. Now stop for a moment and think about your style of living.

Sometimes we ask a woman who wants a long hairdo how many children she has. Based on our own families, we know that mothers are busy people and, generally speaking, don't have much time to spend on their hair. If you want long hair, ask yourself if you have the time for the frequent trims and conditioners that long hair requires. If not, skip it; long, uncared-for hair looks awful. If you're an active person—a sportswoman skiing in the winter and swimming in the summer or a nine-to-five career woman or an all-hours housewife—you should look for a no-fuss haircut and style.

One Last Word . . .

When selecting a hairstyle, you should have a sense of what looks "today." We are not saying that you have to imitate the hairstyles in a trendy, high-fashion magazine. But if you have come along with us this far and then decided to go with a bubble or a beehive, you are off the track. This doesn't mean that if you want height, you can't have it—you can. But today, height comes from the right cut, not from teasing the hair. And it doesn't mean that you cannot wear your hair pulled back into a ponytail—you can. But if you're doing this simply because you think a ponytail is easy, you should know that many of today's styles require less effort than it takes to pull hair back.

Whatever your reasons for wanting to stay with an old style, we guarantee you that there is a new haircut that will give you the shape of that style, except that it will be much easier to handle.

2.

How to Cut Your Own Hair

We were surprised and pleased to learn that a number of our students had been cutting their own hair, some of them for a long time. We imagine that there are many women, and men too, throughout America who cut their own hair and enjoy doing it. Why not—it saves them the expense and time of salon visits. Also, they may feel that no one understands exactly what they want from their hair.

This chapter is for those people who want to cut their own hair, or someone else's. It details all the separate steps necessary to achieve a professional-looking haircut. This chapter is also meant for people who may not want to cut their own hair but who do want to understand what makes a good haircut, so that they can go to a hairdresser equipped with that knowledge.

Granted, haircutting is not something you learn overnight. A professional hairdresser, for example, goes to school for 1,000 to 2,000 hours, and half of that time is spent on learning to cut hair. Then he or she may take advanced haircutting classes.

But it is not necessary for you to have that much practice. If you learn the basic techniques, you can hope to achieve a professional-looking cut each time you pick up the scissors.

Once you have learned how to cut your hair properly, it will reduce the amount of time you spend on your hair. A good cut makes thin hair look thicker, curly hair softer, and lank hair more bouncy. It means disappointment-free hair. With a good cut, hair moves in the right shape so that it will always fall back into place—whether you wet it, shake it, or brush it.

A word of encouragement to anyone who may be slightly apprehensive: of all the novice haircutters we have observed, not one has made an irreparable mistake. Why? Because they were personally involved in what they were doing. It's amazing how cautious you become when you are the one with scissors in hand.

Before we actually show you the step-by-step procedure for cutting hair, we want to talk about the different types of haircutting techniques you can use, give you guidelines for professional results, and make you aware of certain problems you may encounter while cutting. We must also fill you in on the equipment you should have. There is nothing worse than starting a job and learning you don't have the right tools.

Basic Haircuts

We have divided our haircuts into three categories: the blunt cut, the layered cut, and the combination cut (blunt and layers).

The Blunt Cut

The blunt cut refers to a one-length haircut that is achieved by cutting straight across the base of the cut. Most commonly, the blunt cut is executed so that the hair is cut evenly all around the base. It is also possible to use the blunt cut so that hair is longer in the back and shorter on the sides, or shorter in the back and longer on the sides. This kind of cut can be done with just about any hair length from chin to shoulder. It can be very simple or very sophisticated, depending on your choice. The blunt cut offers versatility because you can pull the hair back off your face with combs or barrettes, tie it back with a bow, or wear it straight or turned under. It is also the easiest cut to grow out.

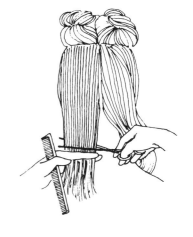

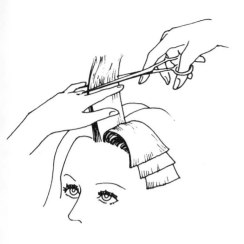

The Layered Cut

The shag is perhaps the most famous example of the layered cut. As the name implies, the hair is cut into layers all over the head. To accomplish this, hair is sectioned off, and each layer is held away from the head and cut anywhere from 1½ to 10 inches, depending on the desired look. Layers are the foundation of all short hairdos. We recommend the layered cut for anyone with curly or frizzy hair because the layers help control the bulk. We also like to see it on fine hair because it gives fullness.

The Combination Cut

The combination cut refers to a blunt cut in back and a layered cut in front to frame the face. Blunt cutting in the back gives body, and layers in the front give softness and movement. The combination cut is the basis for most of today's styles, and we recommend it especially for fine, straight hair as well as wavy hair.

Other Haircuts and Styles

Once you have mastered the blunt and layered cutting techniques and how to combine the two in one cut, you can apply what you have to learned to other areas, such as the following:

Men's hair: See illustrations for two different cuts plus how to trim sideburns or a beard.

Bangs: See illustration for how to cut, keep them in shape, and style them for different facial types.

Long hair: See illustrations for how to give long hair a trim instead of a full cut.

Remember, too, that all the cuts shown are suitable for children's hair. In some cases, you may want to add bangs or modify the length, but cutting children's hair is exactly the same as cutting an adult's, except that it requires more patience.

Several of the haircuts are also suitable for men—for example, the layered cut for short, curly hair on page 41 and the combination cut on page 45.

Twelve Simple Steps to Professional Results in Haircutting

Follow these tips and you will look as if you just came out of an expensive salon.

1. The key to good cutting is precision: cut accurately. Cut a section of hair slowly, snipping with the scissors, never cut a section of hair in one movement. Work with small sections of hair, never with large ones.

2. Pay special attention to the first piece of hair you cut in each section. This piece becomes your guide; all other sections will relate to it.

3. When doing a layered cut, hold the hair you are cutting between your middle and index fingers.

4. When doing a blunt cut, hold hair with your hand flat against your head (and neck), especially in the back.

5. Apply step 4 when cutting bangs.

6. Never cut hair directly over the ear. Comb it either in front of or behind the ear.

7. Allow for hair shrinkage after cutting. Wavy or curly hair may shrink as much as ½ to 1 inch.

8. When combing hair that is to be cut, comb through hair evenly and neatly so that it is not bunched up. Otherwise, an uneven line results.

9. If you are cutting hair directly on the face or neck, use our marker trick: take a face pencil or washable marker and draw in the lines where you should cut. This is virtually mistake-proof (see page 22).

10. Always cut hair *wet* for maximum control.

11. Use a scissors to cut hair, not a razor.

12. Check the cut after you have finished. (We always do.) For a layered cut, do what is called a "cross-check": layers are lifted and checked in the opposite direction from which they have been cut. In other words, if you have cut layers vertically, then you would check them horizontally. After any cut, shake your head from side to side. All the hair should fall back into place.

Special Haircutting Problems

If you follow our step-by-step haircutting instructions, you won't have much trouble cutting your hair. But there are a few problems that even the best professional runs up against.

Cowlick: A cowlick is a strand or section of hair that has a different growth direction from the hair around it, so that it sticks out. When working with a cowlick, allow another inch in length for the cowlick; the extra weight will control it. Judge the rest of your haircut length by that cowlick.

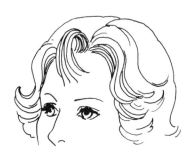

Wave: Allow extra length at the place where the wave is to move into the pattern of the haircut.

Receding hairline: Most people with receding hairlines want to hold on to whatever hair they have, and so they leave it long. Actually, you should cut hair at the temples and center of the forehead shorter, so that the hairline appears more unified.

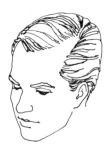 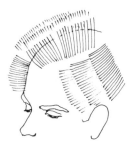 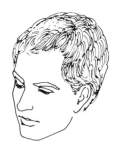

Very thin, sparse hair: If you have barely enough hair to cover your head, stay with a short-to-medium layered cut. Once again, the tendency is to wear this kind of hair too long with the result that the weight of the hair loosens the hair follicles. Cut the hair as shown in the style on page 35 or 41, and keep it soft and brushed toward the face. Also, be sure to handle this kind of hair very gently when cutting.

How to Prepare for a Haircut

Equipment

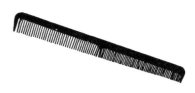

Robe or cutting cape: Wear some kind of comfortable garment such as a T-shirt or other collarless top. Take off all your jewelry, even thin neck chains. Don't place a towel around your neck; let the hair fall, and sweep it up later.

Plastic comb: Use one with wide and fine teeth. You will need this for sectioning and cutting.

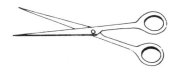

Scissors: These should be 4½-5-inch shears, which should be sharpened every 25 or 30 haircuts. Never use haircutting scissors for any purpose other than cutting hair. (We mainly use Artisan brand scissors).

Hairclips: You will need about 6 clips, which you will use for holding in place the hair that you are not cutting. Plan on 3 short and 3 long clips unless you have particularly long or thick hair, in which case you will need more long ones.

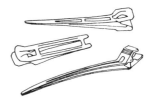

Face pencil or washable marker: For some cuts, we suggest that you mark the lines on your face so you know exactly where to cut.

Mirrors: Stand before a big, clean mirror that is well-lit, such as your bathroom mirror. Place another mirror behind you. We recommend the kind of mirror that can be attached to the wall and turned to any angle. Just make sure that both mirrors are large enough so that you can see everything you are doing.

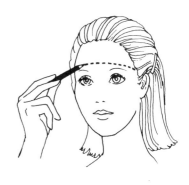

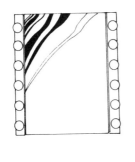

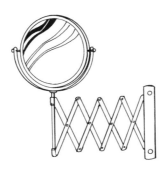

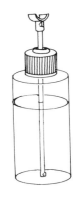

Sprayer: Since hair should be cut wet, have on hand a plant mister or other device that you can spray water, should hair dry while you are cutting.

Psychology

1. Think positively. Remember that you are the one who is controlling the scissors, and you will automatically exercise caution. If it makes you feel more secure, start out with hair trims and progress to full haircuts.

2. Do not cut your hair when you are annoyed or angry. Taking out your frustrations on your hair doesn't work. Besides, your anger will pass a lot more quickly than your hair will grow back in.

3. *Do* cut your hair when you need a general lift of spirit; there is nothing like a new hairstyle to improve your outlook.

Procedure

1. Shampoo your hair at least once—twice if it needs it. Rinse, rinse, rinse, until every last bit of soap is out of your hair.

2. Apply an instant conditioner or cream rinse to your hair by following directions on the label. This is an important step because you must be able to comb through your hair easily.

3. Towel-dry hair slightly—just enough so that it is not dripping.

4. Use the wide-tooth section of your comb to arrange hair into the style you have chosen. If you need to make a part, it must be absolutely clean and straight. Here's how: Comb damp hair back from face. Putting the palm of your hand to your crown on the side you want the part, push hair forward, and your natural part will appear as your hair separates.

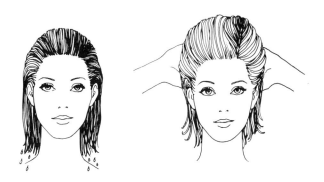

5. Section your hair according to the illustration for each cut. Use hairclips to hold in place the hair you will be working on later.

6. Follow the directions for the haircut you have selected, taking your time and making sure that you understand each step.

Blunt Cut: Even All Around

This cut can be done chin or shoulder length. Cut the hair parted in the middle for the greatest versatility—you can then wear either a center or side part.

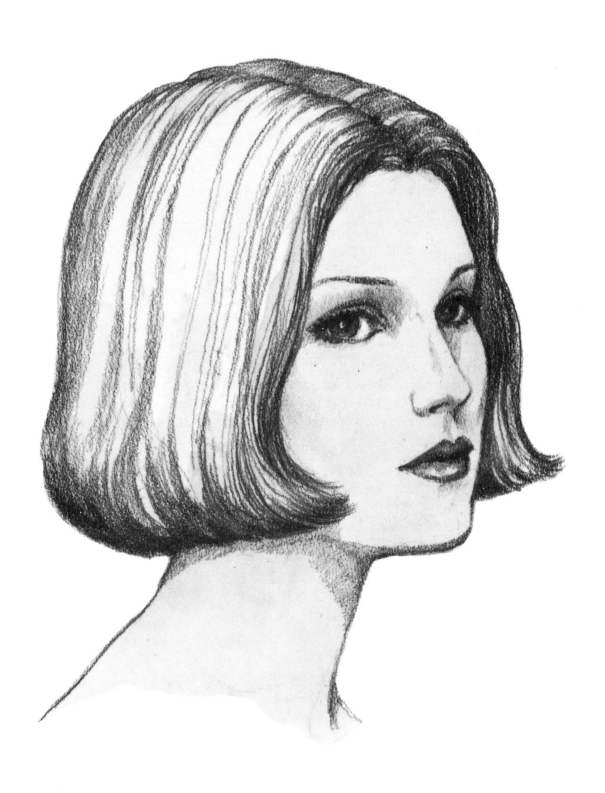

1. Separate back section of hair in half down the middle. Clip one side out of your way. Starting at nape of the neck, bring down a section 2 inches wide by ¾ inch deep. Hold hair firmly with one hand and cut straight across to the desired length. This piece determines the length of your haircut.

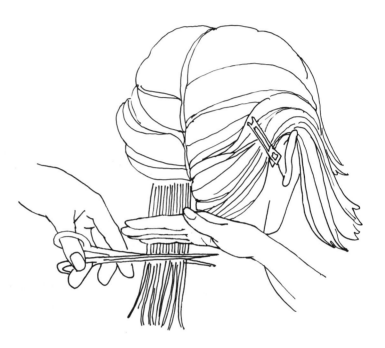

2. Repeat the procedure up to the crown, pulling down the same-size sections and cutting to the length of the first piece. When you have completed one side, do the other.

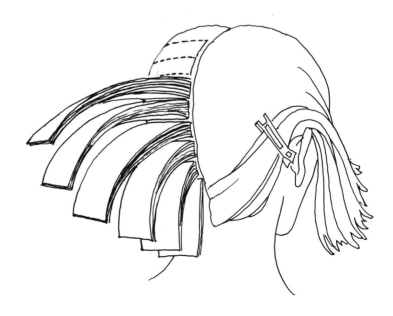

3. If you have very thick hair, you may have to split the back section in quarters—first in half and then in halves again.

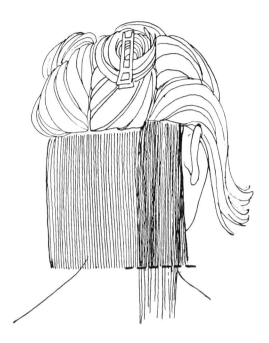

4. Now move on to the sides. Separate a section of hair 1½ inches wide by ½ inch deep and comb down straight *in front of* the ear. Cut straight across so that it is the same length as the back. Continue with the same-size sections up to the part, then repeat the procedure on the other side. *Note:* It is very important that you keep your head straight when you are cutting the sides, otherwise your cut will be uneven.

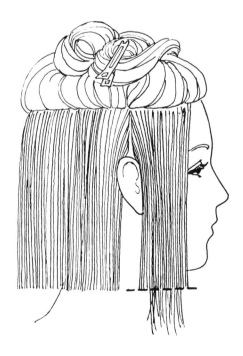

5. Check the line of your haircut when you have finished. It should look like this.

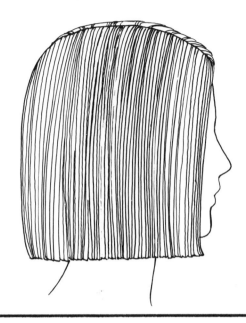

Blunt Cut: Longer in Back, Shorter on Sides

1. Clip hair back from face. Using a face pencil or other water-washable marker, draw a "U-shaped" line from neck to middle of the cheek. This determines the length of your haircut and will serve as your cutting guide. *Note:* If your hair has a slight bend or wave, draw the line slightly lower on the face to allow for hair shrinkage when dry.

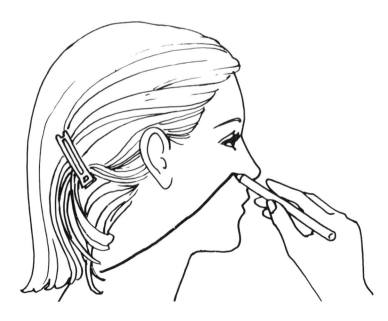

2. Separate hair in front of the ear and pull down sections 1½ inches wide by ½ inch deep. Cut on the line. Using the same-size sections, repeat the procedure up to the part, bringing the hair forward as you cut. Do the same on the other side.

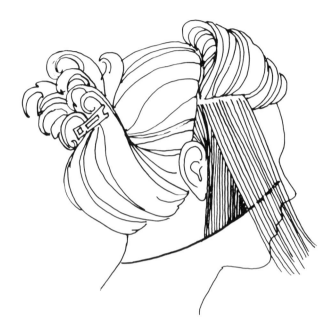

3. Moving behind the ear, separate a section 2 inches wide by ½ inch deep. Comb through and cut on the "U" line you've drawn. Working with the same-size section, repeat procedure up to the part. Do other side.

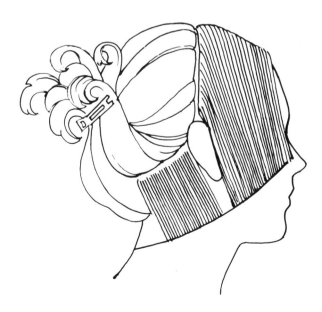

4. Separate back hair in half from crown to nape of neck. Pull down a section 2 inches wide by ¾ inch deep and, holding it down firmly with your hand, cut straight across.

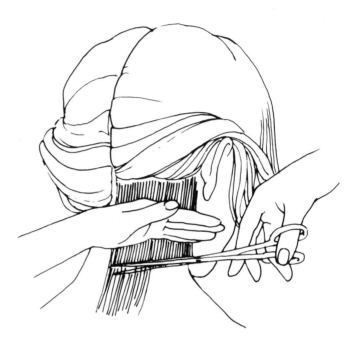

5. Take down the next section of hair, this time 2 inches wide by ½ inch deep, and pull it forward to meet your line. Cut on the line. Repeat the process using the same-size sections up to the crown. Do the same on the other side.

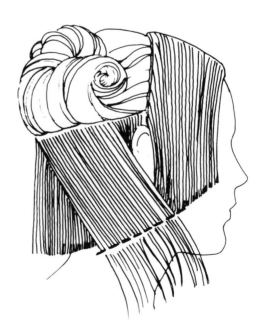

6. This is the shape your hair should have when you have finished.

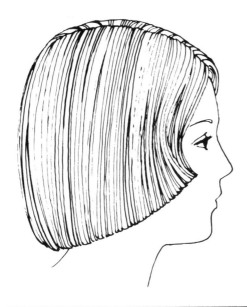

Blunt Cut:
Shorter in Back, Longer on Sides

1. Separate back hair in half down the middle. Working on the diagonal, bring down a section of hair 2 inches wide by ½ inch deep. Holding it down firmly with one hand, cut as though it were part of an inverted "V." This determines the length of your haircut. Continue bringing down the same-size sections on the diagonal until you reach the crown and top of the ear. Repeat process on the other side.

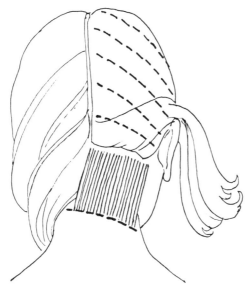

2. To cut side hair and front if you want a pronounced angle: Take a section of hair 1½ inches wide by ½ inch deep from the center part to the ear. Comb it back, and holding it firmly with one hand, cut in to the same inverted "V" as the back. Continue bringing back sections until you reach the front (you will most likely bring back 4-5 sections). Do other side in the same way.

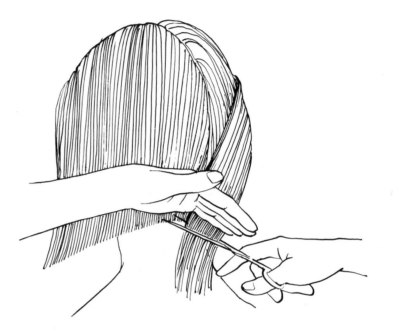

3. To cut side hair and front if you want a less pronounced angle: Take a section of hair 1½ inches wide by ½ inch deep directly above the top of the ear. Cut it on the side to the desired angle. Working with the same-size sections and moving toward the front, pull sections back as shown and then cut.

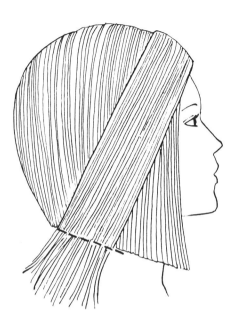

How to Trim Long Hair

Most people with long hair make the mistake of not cutting it often enough—they want as much length as they can get. However, long hair should be *trimmed* every two months; otherwise, you will end up with split ends and broken hair. Here we show how to trim long hair on a "U-shaped" cut—

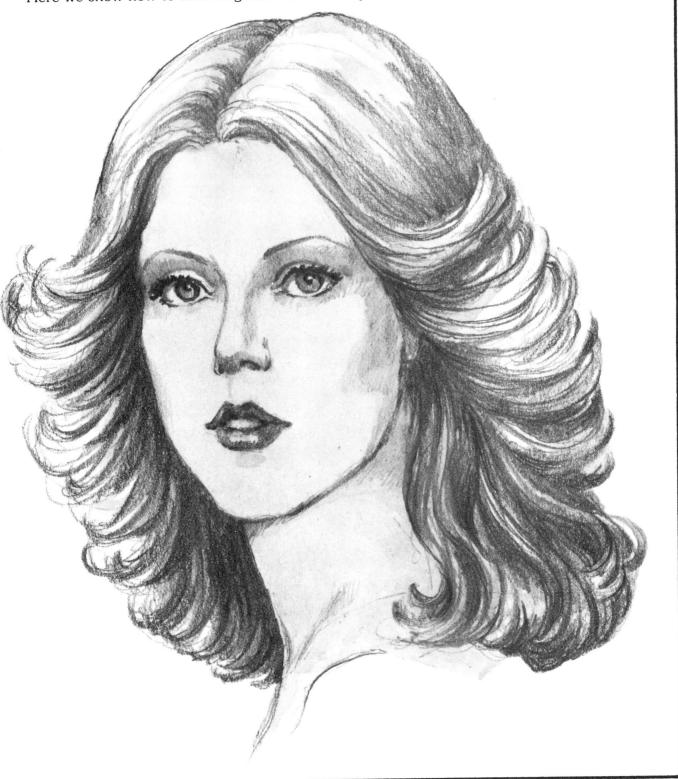

longer in the back and somewhat shorter on the sides. You can also cut long hair blunt all-around (see illustration on page 19), but we like this better because the hair has more movement and will not hang in your face.

1. Separate back hair in half, from crown to nape of neck. Pull down a section of hair 2 inches wide by 1 inch deep and cut straight across at desired length. If you have particularly thick hair, you may have to divide the back hair into additional sections. Repeat procedure up to the crown and then do other side.

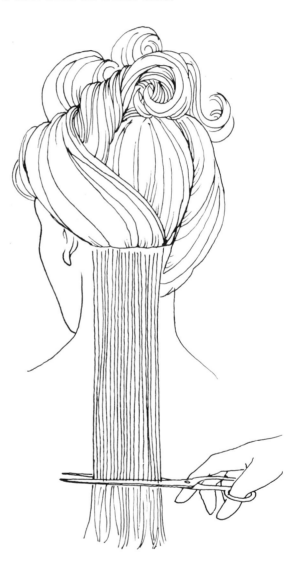

2. Now that you have cut the back straight across, you want to "round out" the hair behind the ears to form the "U." Pull down a section 2 inches wide by 1 inch deep from above and behind the ear, and cut to follow the "U" line. Working with same-size sections, repeat procedure up the part, cutting each section to the same length as the first. Do other side.

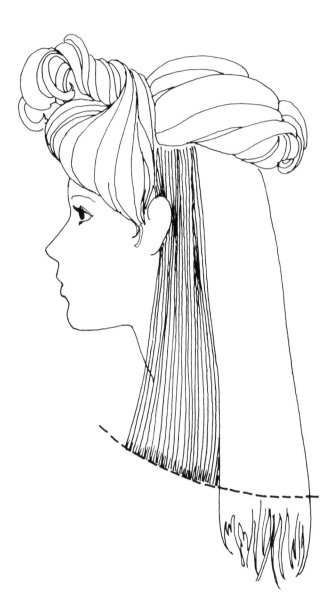

3. Working in front of the ear, separate a section 2 inches wide by 1 inch deep and cut into "U" line. Pull down same-size sections until you reach the part, then repeat procedure on the other side. Make sure you cut all hair while pulled *in front of* the ear, not over it.

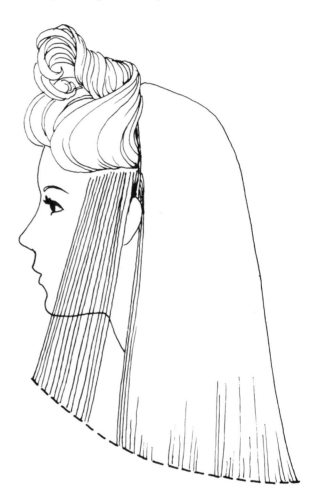

Note: If you want a few layers framing the face on the sides and in front, here's how. Comb all hair in front of the ear forward, then cut an inverted "V" from the sides of the face to mid-nose. Brush back, and you will have slight layers.

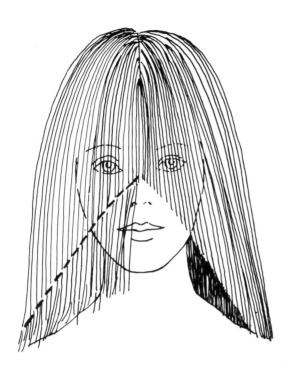

The Layered Cut on Straight Hair

Length: 2½-3 inches all over

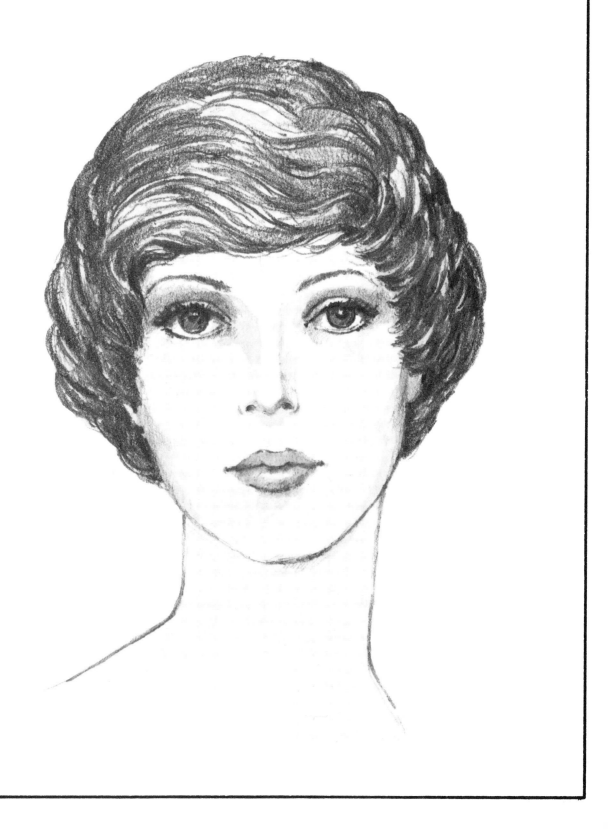

1. Starting at part, take section of hair 1½ inches wide by ½ inch deep and comb straight up. Cut hair to desired length. (*Note:* You are holding hair vertically on the head, so that it is standing straight up, and cutting straight across.) This first piece becomes your guide and establishes the length for the top of the head.

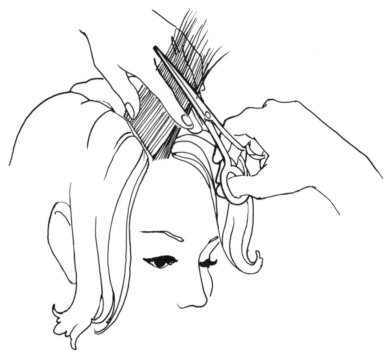

2. Working with the same-size sections, cut entire top from temple to temple and back to crown, as illustrated. At each section, make sure hair is combed through evenly and held out straight from the head.

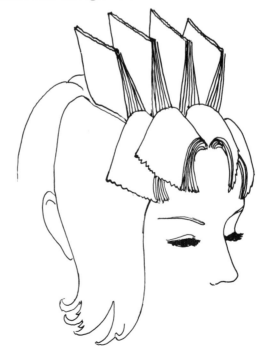

3. Now you are ready to do the sides. Starting at the part, take a 1½-inch-wide by ½-inch-deep section on the diagonal and comb down on the face. Take a small section of hair that has been cut on top, near the part, and pull down on the forehead. Side hair should be cut to the same length as this piece and should conform to the same angle.

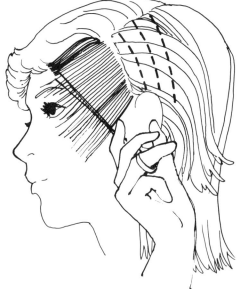

4. Continue bringing down same-size sections, working on the diagonal toward the crown. But only the first section is cut on the face; the remaining sections should be cut held in the air. This is what gives hair the layered effect. By the

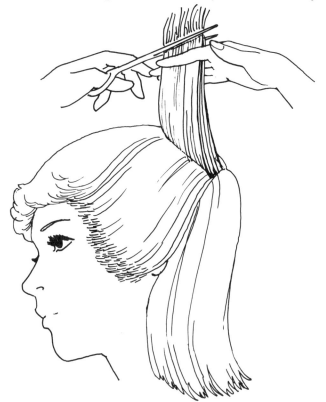

time you reach the crown, your side hair should be taking this shape. Repeat the procedure on other side.

5. Separate back in half down the middle. Starting at the part and at the crown, pull out a section of hair 3 inches wide by ¾ inch deep and hold it out from the head at a 45-degree angle. Cut to same length as top section on the crown. Work toward the ear, then go back to the other side and repeat the procedure. Illustration indicates how hair should look when cut on the left, and hair on right side being cut at the nape of the neck.

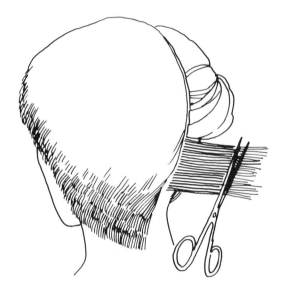

6. Check the cut. Go back over all the layers and pull them out from the head to make sure they are even. If not, you may have to do a little snipping here and there.

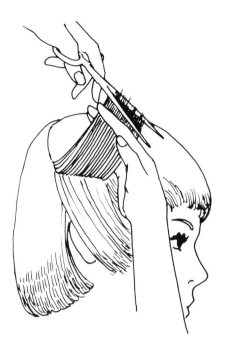

The Layered Cut on Curly or Permanent Waved Hair

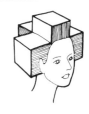

Length: 2-4 inches all over the head. *Tip:* Curly hair shrinks when dry, so leave an extra ¾ inch. Always hold the hair away from the head while cutting, almost as if hair were being cut in a box formation. See illustration for the line of the cut, which you should keep in mind. For the greatest accuracy, work with small sections.

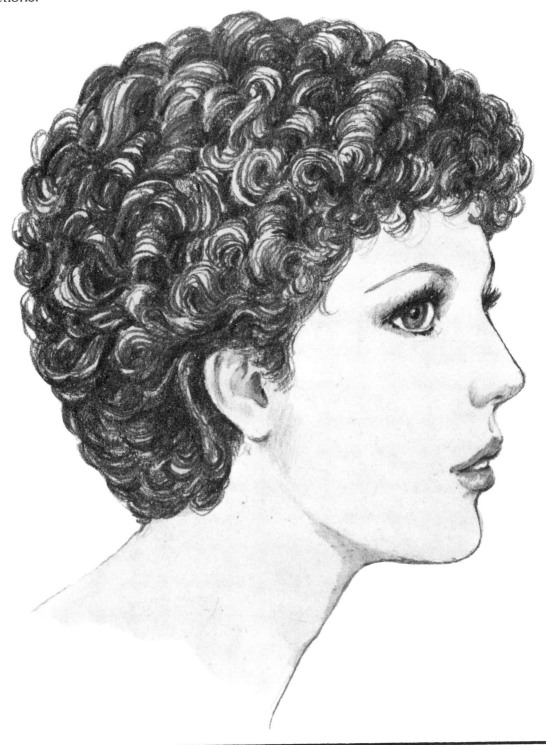

1. Starting at the part or at the temple, comb out a section of hair 1½ inches wide by ½ inch deep. Cut vertically on the head, that is, from front to back.

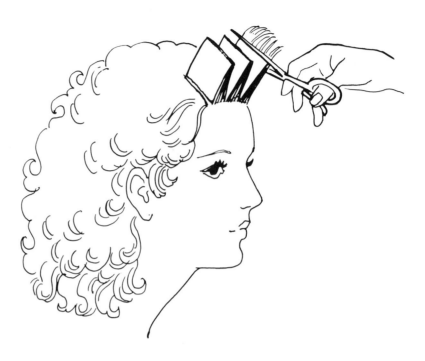

2. Working with same-size sections, cut from temple to temple and back to the crown, always holding hair straight up.

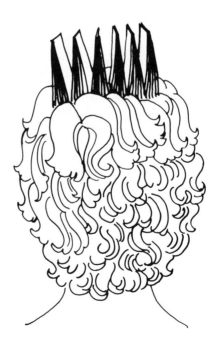

3. Go back to the part where you started and pull up the first piece of top hair that you cut. Now pull out a side section 1½ inches long by ½ inch deep and cut it to the same length as your first piece. Continue procedure to the ear, then do the other side. Only cut the hair that is in front of the ear.

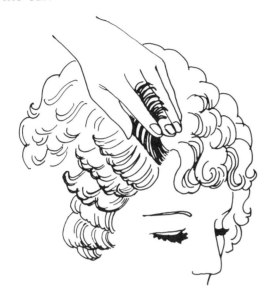

4. Separate back hair in half from crown to nape of neck. Starting at the crown and at the part, pull out section of hair 1½ inches by ½ inch, and cut vertically as indicated in sketch. Work with same-size sections and move toward back of ear. Back should be cut same length as the top hair on the crown.

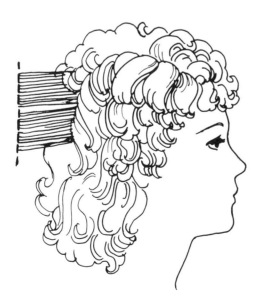

Combination Cut: Blunt All Over, Layered Look When Swept Back

This is often called the "bowl cut." See the illustration for the silhouette of the cut. This versatile cut can be worn in a

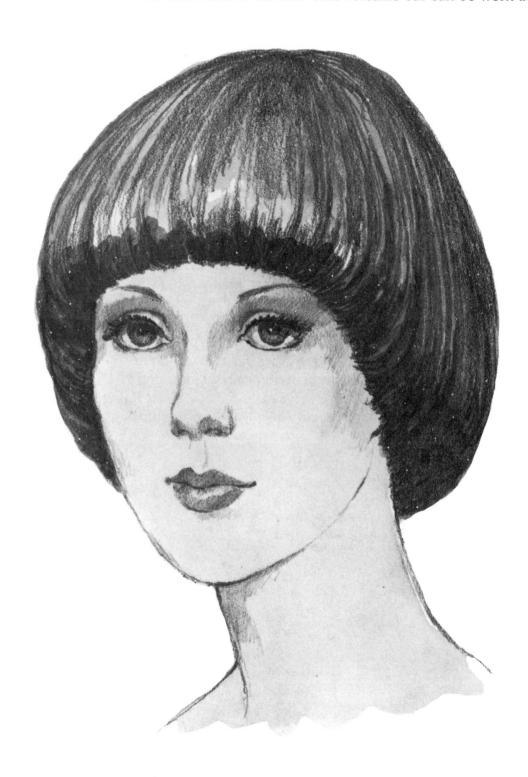

variety of ways, and you can cut it anywhere from chin to
collarbone length.

1. Starting at front, by the temple, bring out a piece of hair 1½ inches wide by ½ inch deep. Cut as shown, but cut hair ¼ to ½ inch longer than you want it. This piece now becomes your guide, and all other pieces in the front should be cut to this length. *Note:* If you have very fine hair, cut this piece right on your forehead, not pulled out.

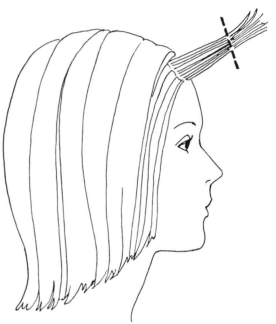

2. Divide hair in front from the top of one ear to top of the other ear; clip rest of hair back. Starting at the ear, bring forward sections 1½ inches wide by ½ inch deep and cut to the length of the first piece and so that it conforms to the bowl silhouette.

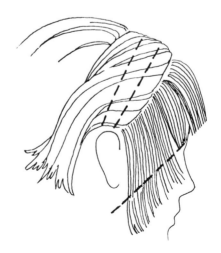

3. Continue cutting, moving from one side to the other. Hair should fall as illustrated. Remember, if hair is thick, cut straight out; if fine, cut on the head.

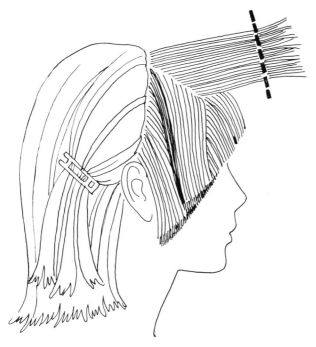

4. Separate back in half down the middle. Starting at nape of neck, pull down section 2 inches wide by ½ inch deep. Hold hair down firmly with your hand and cut straight across at desired length. Repeat procedure with same-size sections going up toward the crown. Do the same on other side.

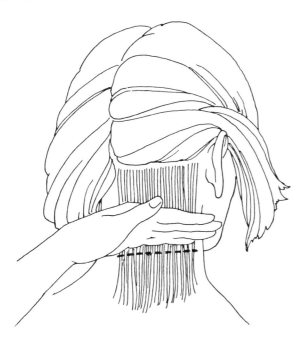

5. Now you must join the cut at the sides and back together. Take a 2-inch-wide section directly behind the ear and comb it down, clipping bulk of hair from the crown back. Cut hair so that you round off the corner, once again following the bowl silhouette.

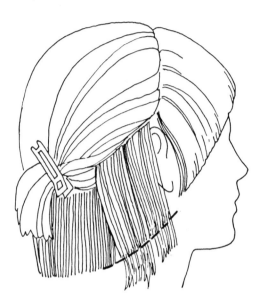

6. Repeat the process sectioning diagonally to the top of the head. Do the same on the other side.

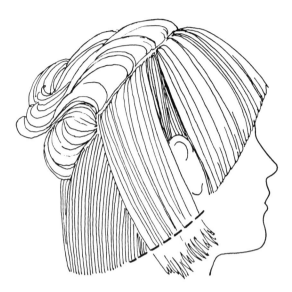

Combination Cut: Layered on Top and Sides, Blunt in Back

Length can be anywhere from chin to collarbone. Study the silhouette of the cut before starting.

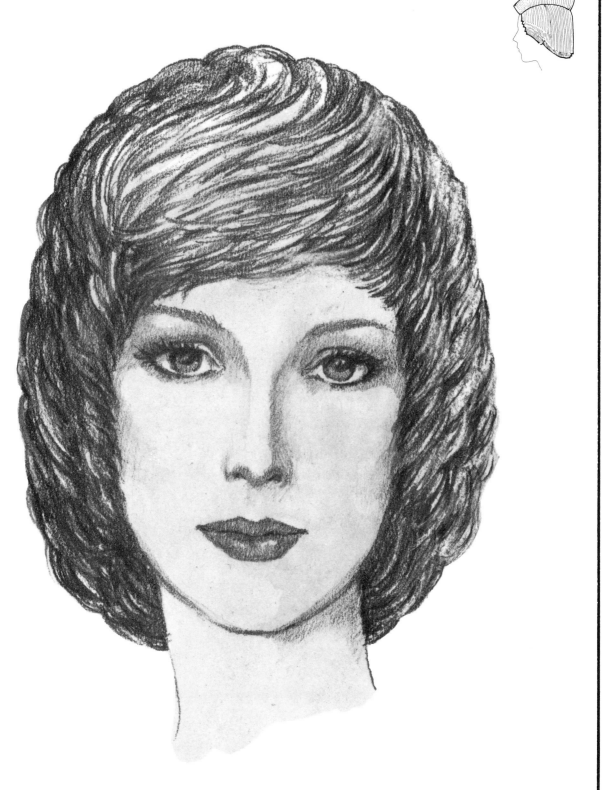

1. To establish length for hair that will frame the face, pull down a section from the top front, 2 inches across and ½ inch deep. Hold hair down firmly on forehead and cut straight across about ½ inch below the eyebrow.

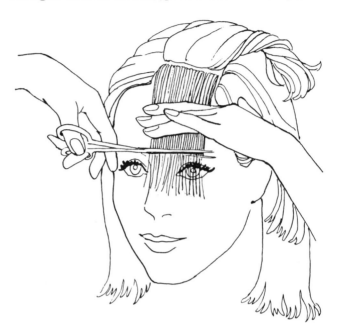

2. Starting at the part or at the temple, take a 1½-inch-wide by ½-inch-deep section of hair and comb straight up. Using the hair you just cut as your guide for length, cut the hair in this section the same length.

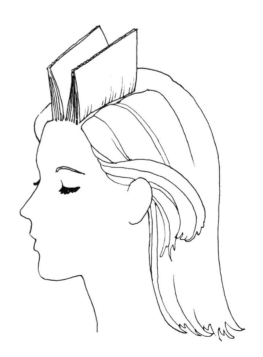

3. Continue with the same-size sections, cutting all the hair from the front of the face to the top of the ear. Do the other side.

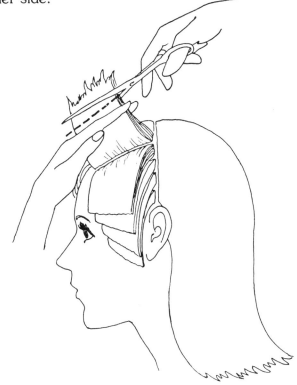

4. When you have finished cutting the sides, comb them forward on the face. They may need to be evened out slightly.

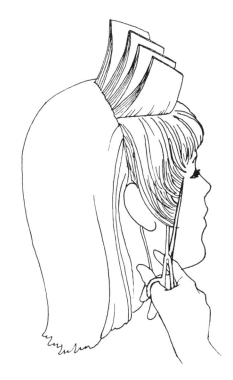

5. Separate back hair down the middle. Starting at the nape of the neck, pull down a section of hair 2 inches wide by ½ inch deep. Hold hair down firmly with one hand and cut straight across at desired length.

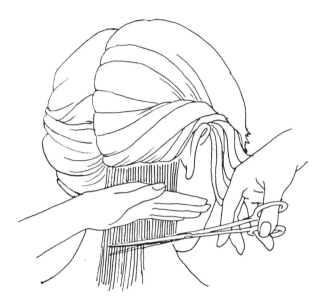

6. Continue pulling down same-size sections of hair, moving toward the crown. Repeat this process on the other side. *Note:* If your hair is very thick, you may have to divide the back in half, once again.

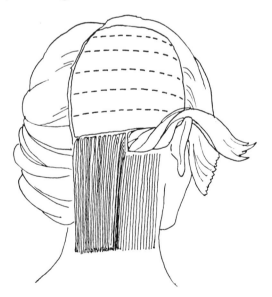

7. Steps 7-9 show you how to achieve the rounded angle where sides meet the front of the silhouette. Take a 2-inch-wide by ½-inch-deep section of hair directly behind the ear and pull it toward the face. Cut to conform with the same line as the front.

8. Continue upward toward the crown, working with 2-inch by ½-inch sections, pulling hair toward the face and cutting.

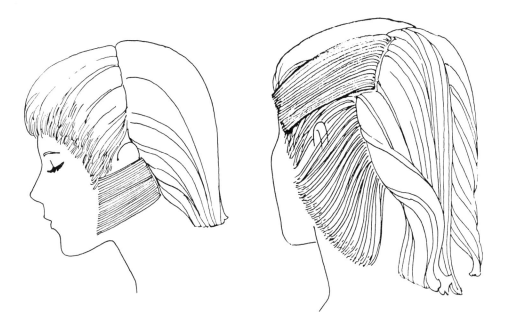

9. Continue making sections from neck to crown working toward the middle of the back. Repeat procedure with the other side.

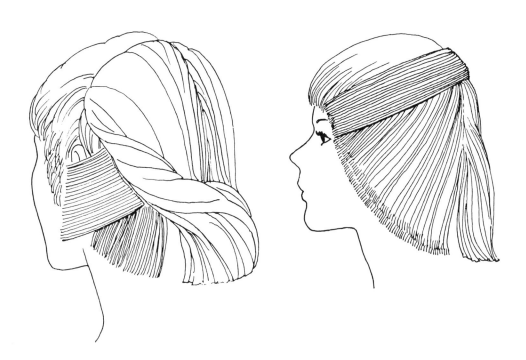

Combination Cut:
Layered Front and Sides, Blunt Back

Length can be anywhere from chin to collarbone.

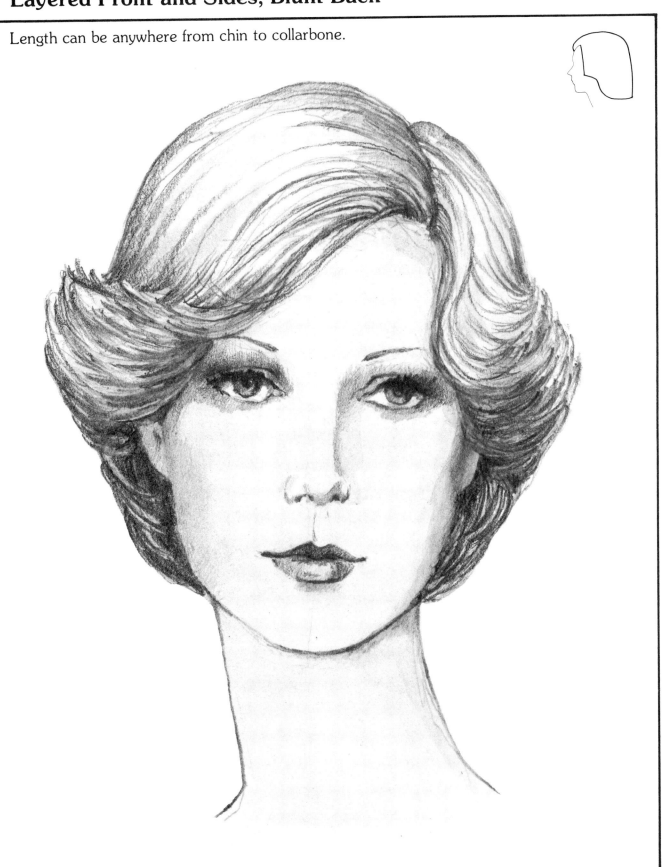

1. Starting on the side opposite the part, divide hair in front of the ear. Bring down a section of hair 1½ inches wide by ½ inch deep. Cut hair at angle shown to desired length.

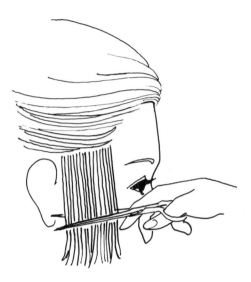

2,3. Continue bringing down same-size sections, cutting at the same angle and length.

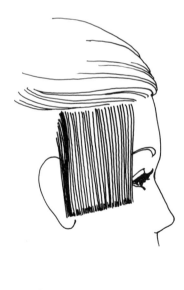

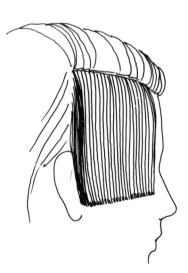

4. As you approach the top, there will be more hair to cut, so make sure to cut it at the same angle.

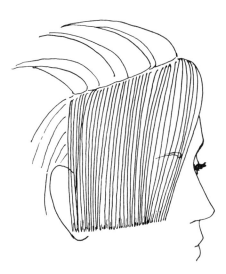

5. When you have finished one side, comb hair back. It should look like this.

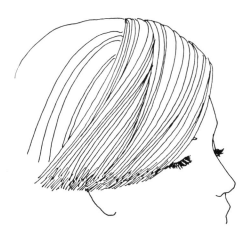

6. Go to the other side, bringing hair down in 1½-inch-wide by ½-inch-deep sections. Cut at the same angle as the first side. *Note:* If your hair is thick, you may have to divide hair into two sections.

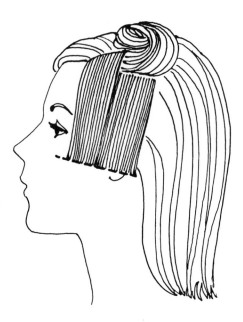

7. Separate back hair in half. Bring down section of hair 1½ inches wide by ½ inch deep. Hold hair down firmly with one hand and cut straight across at desired length.

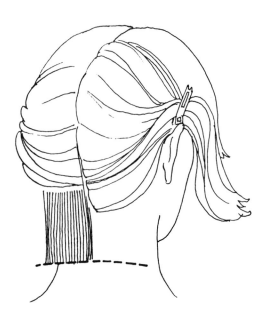

8. Working with same-size sections, continue cutting up to crown, so that hair looks like this. Repeat procedure on other side. Silhouette illustrates general outline.

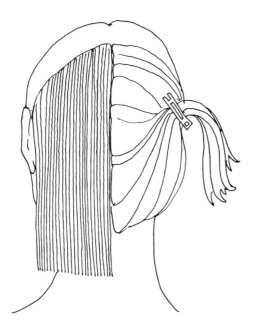

9. Steps 9-11 show you how to angle the sides to the front. Directly behind the ear, take a diagonal section 2 inches wide by ¾ inch deep, pull forward, and cut so that it conforms to line of silhouette illustrated.

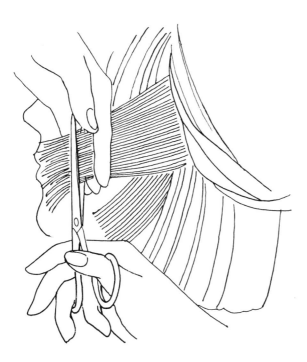

10. Continue pulling same-size sections toward face and cutting.

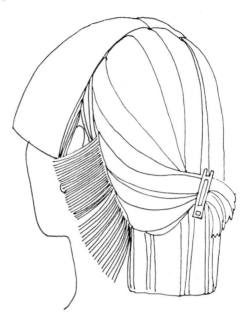

11. Using diagonal sections, continue process until you reach center back part. Repeat procedure with other side.

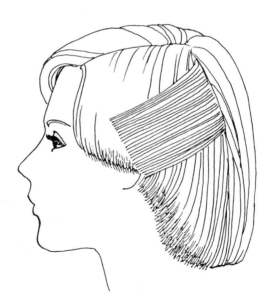

12. When you are finished, check the cut. Hair combed back
should look like this.

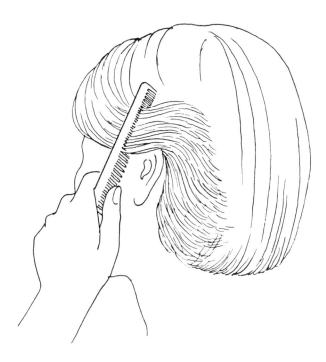

The Right Way to Cut Bangs

Cutting bangs isn't hard, but it is not a matter of chopping a straight line across the forehead, either. The secret to good bang cutting is bringing the hair down in sections . . . and then cutting each section *individually*. Also, you must allow for hair shrinkage. On curly hair, for example, you should allow an extra ½ inch. On straight hair, bangs stay pretty much the same length, but if you are ever in doubt, allow more length than you think right.

BANG TIPS FOR DIFFERENT FACES

Round face: light, wispy bangs
Long face: long, wide bangs
Square face: wispy bangs swept to the side
Heart-shaped face: wide, rounded bangs brushed to the side
Triangle face: light, wispy bangs
Diamond face: rounded bangs, medium thickness

1. Pull all hair back and divide section for bangs.

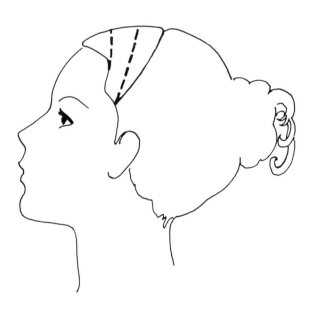

2. Split section in half exactly, as if you were making a center part. Starting on one side, pull down a small section of hair and comb through so that it is perfectly smooth. *Hold it down firmly on the forehead and cut across in small, snipping motions.*

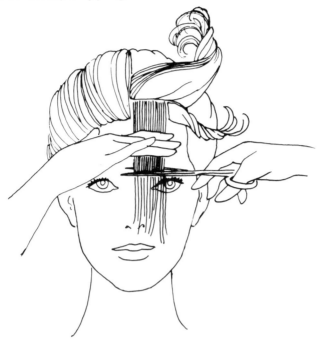

3. Bring down next section and comb through with the first section you have cut. Hold down on the forehead and cut across. Repeat procedure until you finish one side, then move on to the other.

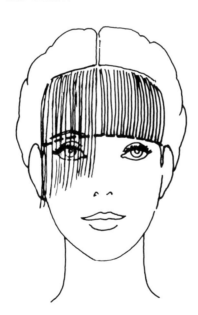

Men's Hair: How to Cut Curly Hair and How to Trim a Beard

All hair is cut in layers, about 1½ to 2 inches. At every step, hair is cut while held out from the head, similar to the illustration for step 6. After you have finished, go back over the cut and make sure that all layers are of equal length; this is important if the hair is to fall into its own natural shape.

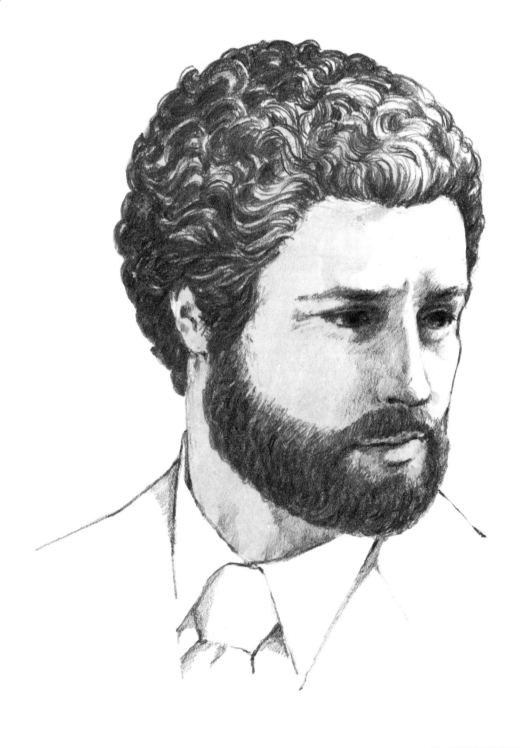

1. Bring down on the forehead a section of hair 1½ inches wide by ½ inch deep. Cut to desired length, allowing ¾ inch for shrinkage. Hold this piece of hair straight up and, using it as a guide for length, cut the entire top of the head, from temple to temple and back to crown, cutting all the hair the same length as your first piece. You will be cutting hair vertically, holding the scissors from front to back.

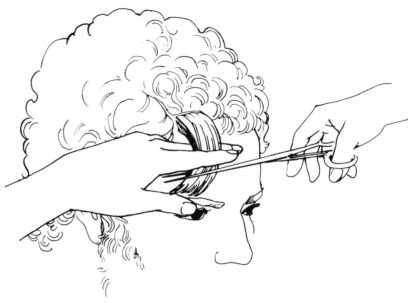

2. Starting at the side part or at the temple, separate section of hair 1½ inches wide by ½ inch deep. Once again, this piece should be the same length as the first piece you cut. Cut both sides, holding each section out from the head as you cut.

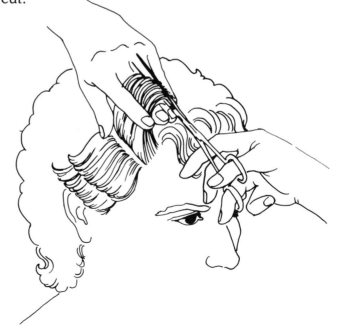

3. Separate a piece of hair from the crown, which you have already cut. This piece determines the length for your back hair.

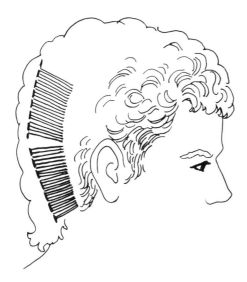

4. To cut hair from crown to nape of neck, take sections 1½ inches by ½ inch and, pulling them straight out, cut to the same length as crown piece. Cut all hair from either side of middle back to ears.

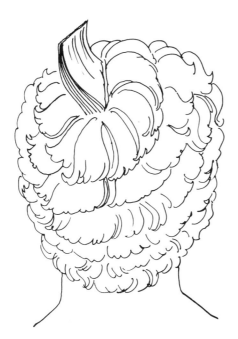

5. Although you have now cut the entire head, you need to reframe some hair around the ear. Take a section 1½ inches wide by ½ inch deep behind the ear, pull forward and cut. Repeat this procedure on other side.

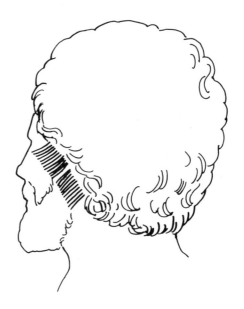

6. *To Trim Beard:* A beard is cut in layers. Comb through the hair in the opposite direction from which it grows, and cut each layer so that all layers are even. For best control, use either a comb or your fingers. Beards should be trimmed to a length of ½ to ¾ of an inch.

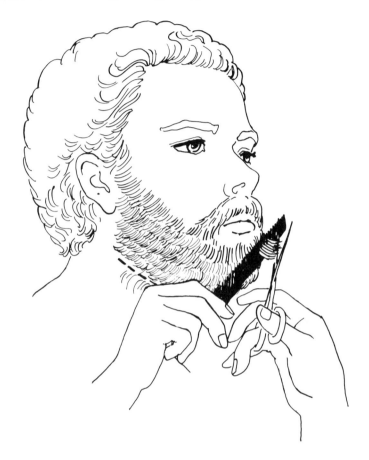

Men's Hair: How to Cut Straight Hair and How to Trim a Sideburn

This is a layered cut for men, meant to be worn anywhere from 2-3 inches long. The silhouette illustrates that all hair is cut the same length.

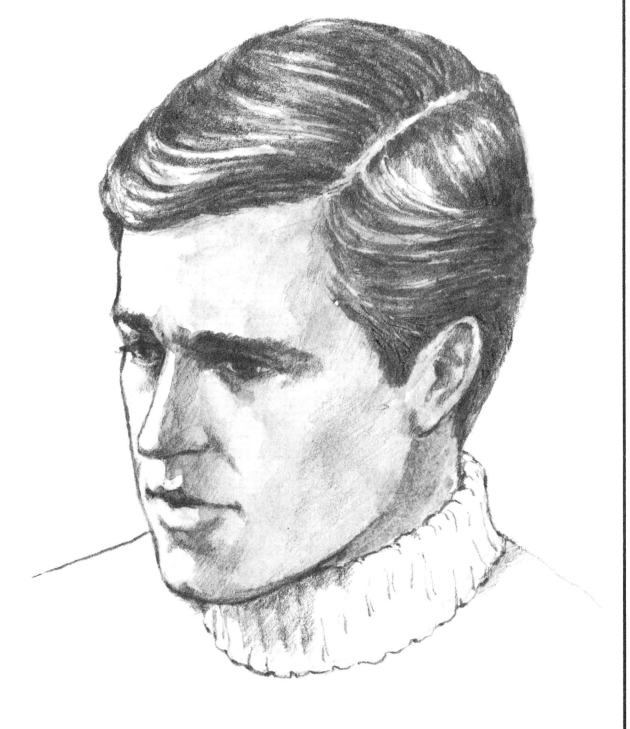

1.   Start at the side of the part. To shape a sideburn, comb through and snip at an angle to desired length.

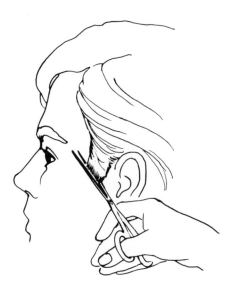

2.   Starting at the sideburn, bring down sections 1½ inches wide by ½ inch deep and cut at the same angle.

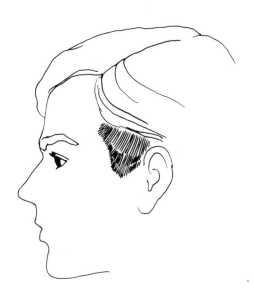

3. Working up toward the part, bring down same-size sections and cut the same length. Repeat procedure two more times, working from the ear up to the part. Do the same on the other side, but cut *only* up to the temple.

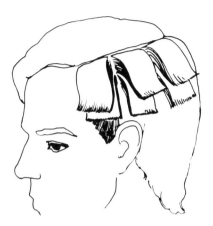

4. Separate back hair in half, from the nape of the neck to the crown. Starting at the part, bring forward a section 1½ inches wide by ½ inch deep. Repeat procedure, working forward toward the back of the ear. Continue on next level until all hair is cut on one side of back part. Repeat procedure with the other side.

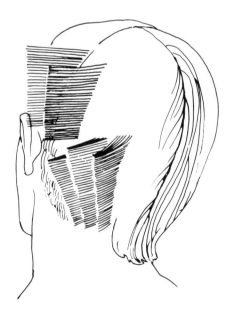

5. Go to the top section. Starting at the front and at the part, separate a section 1½ inches wide by ½ inch deep. Holding it straight up, cut the hair so that it is the same length as the hair cut previously at the temple. The top should be cut in 4 sections across from temple to temple and 2 sections deep to crown, as illustrated.

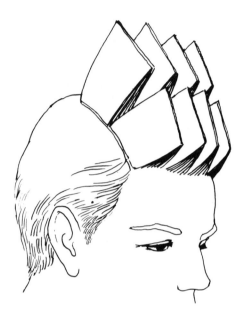

3.

Today's Look and How to Get It

When you look at old photographs, the clothes immediately tell you the decade in which the picture was taken. So do the hairstyles. There's no mistaking a Victorian "Gibson Girl," a '20s bob, a '40s pageboy, or a '50s bubble. Today's look in hair is equally distinctive; styles are natural, carefree, and swinging. The texture and general appearance of hair is natural. It's a must for hair to look healthy and shiny. Gone are the days when you could hide sick or damaged hair under teasing or hair spray. Today's hair tells all.

What does your hair say about you? Does it look well-maintained? Do you follow a regular program of care? What about the style—are you treating your hair properly so that it keeps its line throughout the day?

It is not hard to achieve the current look—in fact, it is probably easier to have a "with it" hairstyle now than it ever was. But you must understand the components that go into that look.

Hair Health

If you want your hair to look attractive, the first thing you need is a good haircut. The next important factor is your hair's condition—its shine, its bounce, its resiliency. The right shampoos and conditioners are crucial.

Most women think they know all there is to know about shampooing. At various times we have asked both students and clients to give us a demonstration of how they wash their hair. Most women are amused by the request. As one woman said: "I've been shampooing my hair for years. What could you possibly teach me?" As it turned out, the answer to that question was: "A great deal!" She, along with just about everyone else, skipped lightly over the *most important part* of a shampoo—the rinse. Just because the suds are no longer visible, that does not necessarily mean that all the shampoo is out. If you do not rinse enough, you will leave a film on your hair, which will dull it. Also, hair with shampoo in it may be difficult to cut and will not take a good blow dry or set.

About Shampooing

First, let's clear up a myth once and for all: frequent shampooing does not mean your hair will fall out or become weaker or lighter in color. On the other hand, if you don't shampoo often enough, oil that is allowed to accumulate on the scalp will give off an unpleasant odor and can also lead to infection, in addition to spoiling your appearance. So please, wash your hair as often as necessary, which means as soon as it loses bounce and shine. For some people this may be every three days; for others, it may mean *every day!*

What Kind of Shampoo?

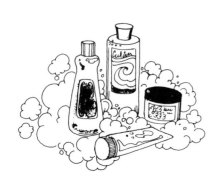

One key to proper shampooing is to know which product is best for you. There are several ways to find out: ask a hairdresser, go to a large drugstore and read over the labels, or send away for trial samples. Keep switching until you find a shampoo that you are happy with. A good shampoo should leave your hair clean and manageable and not irritate your scalp. We personally like protein- or oil-based shampoos; they seem to work best for most people.

Here are some guidelines to help you choose a shampoo for your hair type:

Normal hair: If your hair still looks fresh several days after shampooing, use a shampoo formulated for normal or regular hair.

Oily hair: People with oily hair usually have no problem in recognizing the fact—their hair feels greasy a day or so after they wash it. It is a problem that occurs often with fine hair. If your hair is fine and oily, alternate an oily shampoo with a regular one or with a protein shampoo. If your hair is thick and oily, then always use an oily hair formula.

Dry hair: If your hair is flyaway, and electricity seems to spark when you brush, choose a dry hair shampoo with conditioning formula.

Limp and fine hair: If your hair never seems to have enough body, try a body-building shampoo with an egg or protein formula.

Chemically treated hair: Protect hair that has been chemically treated with a special shampoo for this hair type.

Dandruff: There are many medicated and tar shampoos on the market that are helpful in correcting dandruff. It is a matter of finding one with the ingredients that are best for you. If you have stubborn dandruff (or suspect it might be something more serious), go to a doctor for a prescription shampoo.

Gray hair: Gray hair has a tendency to be coarse and dry. Use shampoo recommended for dry hair.

Dull hair: If hair is not shiny, it can be due to a variety of reasons (see p. 92). Certain shades of ash-brown hair usually look dull; if that's your problem, try a highlighting shampoo. (*Note:* this is not meant to be an easy way out for neglected hair.)

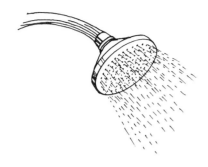

Dry shampoos are good to have around for emergencies, but they are not meant for regular use—nothing takes the place of good shampooing. Dry shampoos are basically powder formulas that you spray on the hair to absorb dirt. Brushing out the powder is a little difficult if you have thick hair, but the end result will be cleaner-looking hair.

Once you have chosen your shampoo, you need a good strong shower or spray attachment. We know that many people wash their hair in a basin, using a pitcher of water to rinse. This is probably the least effective way to get hair clean. Without the strength of a spray, you won't be able to get all the soap out. And as we have already stated, the result is dull hair.

Ten Steps To A Professional Shampoo

1. Either brush your hair or give yourself a fast (2- to 3-minute) massage to loosen dirt. Make sure that there are no snarls or tangles in the hair.

2. Read the label on the shampoo bottle for any special instructions. For example, some manufacturers suggest that you leave the shampoo on for five minutes to derive the best benefits.

3. Pour some shampoo into the palm of your hand and dilute with a few drops of water. (This is especially important if you have thin or limp hair.)

4. Work shampoo into scalp. Then massage all over with fingertips, not your nails. (*Note:* Don't expect a great deal of lather from protein shampoos; they contain few, if any, detergents.)

5. Once you've gone over the scalp thoroughly, move toward the hair ends. Always move from the scalp to the ends, not against the grain.

6. Rinse hair thoroughly with lukewarm water, then finish off with a cool rinse. When rinsing, pay special attention to the area near the ears and all around the hairline.

7. Follow up your shampoo with a conditioner, using it according to the label instructions.

8. Wrap hair in a terrycloth towel to blot up excess water. Do not wring out hair or rub it with the towel. Wet hair stretches like an elastic band and is very easily broken.

9. To comb out hair, use a plastic wide-tooth comb. Never brush through wet hair—you'll break it. You should not

have any snarls if you have used a conditioner, but if
snarls occur, work from the bottom up, using one hand to
press your hair against your scalp as you work on the
ends.

10. Dry hair naturally or with a blow dryer.

About Conditioners

Hair conditioners are as essential to the hair as moisturizers
are to the skin. They are a key part of your hair-care program.

A good conditioner should:

detangle hair and make it more manageable

reduce frizzies

make hair less flyaway

add shine

add body

There are many conditioners on the market and women
often assume that they all do the same thing. They don't! To
have beautiful hair, you must zero in on the conditioner that
best fits your particular hair problem.

Generally, conditioners fall into one of two categories:
instant or deep conditioning. An instant conditioner should be
used after every shampoo, especially if you blow-dry your hair.
Left on for only five minutes, an instant conditioner coats your
hair and thus protects it. A deep-penetrating conditioner, on
the other hand, does a much bigger job. Left on for thirty
minutes, it penetrates the shaft so that the hair holds moisture,
seals up any cracks in the hair's cuticles, and makes hair more
resistant to breakage.

We recommend a deep-penetrating conditioner for everyone
at least once a month, more often for those with very dry,
broken, or processed hair. When deep-conditioning your hair,
wrap a towel around your head and sit under a dryer for the
prescribed time. This is what we do in the salon to achieve
optimum results.

Chart 3 (see p. 82) lists hair conditioners suitable for various
types of hair.

Chart 3. Hair Conditioners

Conditioner Type	Hair Type
Hairdressing cream protects fragile hair from the elements and helps combat dry ends. Use sparingly. *Examples:* Alberto VO-5, Clairol's Vitapointe	Good for dry hair, especially in winter. Also suggested for hair that lacks luster or is prone to split ends.
Cream rinses remove snarls and tangles for easier combing. Apply after shampoo and rinse out. *Examples:* Redken's Phinal Phase, Breck's Cream Rinse	Use on long hair, children's hair, or any hair type that snarls easily.
Instant conditioner is a 5-minute treatment used after shampoo. Rinse out. Detangles hair, provides body, adds shine. *Examples:* Revlon's Flex, Redken's Climatress	For every hair type except fine. Oily hair types should use only on ends.
Deep-penetrating conditioner treats dry, damaged, or chemically processed hair. Restores shine and body by sealing up rough edges of the hair shaft. *Examples:* Clairol's Condition Beauty Pack Treatment, Wella's Kolestral	Excellent for all hair types once a month. Essential for very dry, overprocessed hair. Can be used as often as once a week.
Hot-oil treatment *Examples:* Ogilvie's Recon- ditioning Hot Oil Treatment	Hot-oil treatment should be used on dry, brittle hair only.

Some people are reluctant to use a conditioner because they fear it will make their hair dirtier faster. To some degree this is true: a conditioner coats your hair shaft; and as a result, you may find that your hair feels somewhat oily. But when you think about air pollution, blow dryers, electric curlers, smoke, and all the other things that can attack your hair, doesn't it make sense to use a good conditioner for protection? We have found one way to eliminate that oily problem is to use less conditioner than the manufacturer recommends. If your hair is of medium length or shorter, or if it is finer than average hair, you can easily do with less than the recommended amount. Conditioners are not a case of "if one dose is good, two must be better!"

Conditioners to Avoid

Now that we have gone on about how wonderful conditioners are for your hair and told you what we like, we will also give you the other side of the story. We are against conditioners that do not rinse out. As a rule, these conditioners are called "body builders," and they are meant to add volume to the hair and help hold a set. Too often, these body builders leave a dull film on the hair and make the scalp flaky. If you are using one of these to hold the line of your style—forget it. A good cut or permanent can do a better job.

Other Conditioners

Chart 3 gives you the names of some commercial preparations that we like. But many of our clients have asked if we have any special conditioning formulas. We do have one that we used in our native Italy. It is our special formula, and it has been featured in such magazines as *Vogue, Harper's Bazaar,* and *Mademoiselle,* among others. We feel that it is superb for all hair types, and we especially recommend it for hair that has been chemically treated. Chemicals destroy the hair's sugar bond. Our formula helps to restore this sugar bond and give you the shiniest, healthiest hair ever.

Nardi's Special Blackstrap Molasses Treatment

For medium length hair, mix 2 tablespoons blackstrap molasses with 2 tablespoons Redken's Climatress. Apply generously, section by section, to the hair and scalp. Wrap head tightly in a terrycloth towel and sit under a dryer for 30 minutes. Rinse out formula thoroughly under lukewarm water for 2 to 5 minutes. The result: hair that's manageable, glossy, and alive.

Hair Exercises

Brushing

We love the old movie scene where the glamorous star, swathed in a luxurious dressing gown, is sitting at a vanity brushing her hair. We suspect that for most women, ritual hairbrushing has gone the way of satin robes and dressing tables, which is unfortunate. Because a good hairbrushing is the cheapest way to give your hair extra luster and build up a real gloss. It is also the best way to distribute oils to the hair ends. Regularly brushed hair feels silky and soft and smooth and polished.

What kind of brush should you buy? There's a good deal of controversy over natural vs. nylon bristle, both sides having their champions. Personally, we feel that when it comes to brushing for gloss, natural bristle is the answer; when you're using a brush for styling, a nylon bristle is more effective.

If you have extremely fragile or damaged hair, do not brush it until it is back in shape. But for normal hair, a regular program of brushing is what makes the difference in hair appearance. So, please, don't take a few random swipes and feel that you have done some good.

First, sit down in a chair to brush your hair—you'll last longer. Hang your head down. Draw the brush through the full length of the hair, working from the nape of the neck to the forehead. Make sure that you return the brush to the scalp and the neck after each long stroke. Do this for fifty or so strokes. It takes only three to five minutes—not a very big investment when it pays off so well.

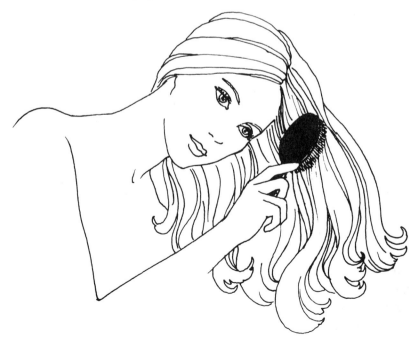

Massage

Scalp massage is one of our favorite hair exercises because it can be fit into anyone's schedule. Massage while you are talking on the phone, resting, or watching TV. Done properly, massage will make your scalp tingle, improve circulation, and stimulate hair growth. If you have a tight scalp, which not only feels unpleasant but can also lead to hair loss, massage is especially important. As one ages, massage should be more frequent because circulation is apt to decline.

Give yourself a massage at home the way we do it in the salon: Starting in the front, take a section of hair about the size you would wind around a roller; then, placing your fingers one inch from the scalp, pull gently. Take another section and repeat the maneuver until you have covered the entire head. To finish off, use the fat pads of your fingers to rub scalp vigorously. Your scalp will tingle!

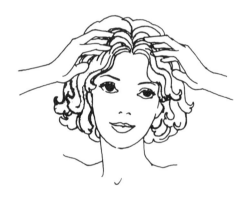

Other Exercises

Anything that revs up the circulation is good for the hair. If you can do it, stand on your head—a trick used by models for a glowing cover-girl look. Or take up yoga, which stimulates the circulation because it is such a wonderful way to ease tension.

Hair Problems

As we said before, few people have perfect hair. Conditioning and correct shampooing can go a long way to help you achieve today's look of shining, healthy hair. But certain hair problems can prevent you from getting *the look*. What follows is a list of various trouble areas—how to recognize them, what causes them, and what you can do to correct them.

Oily Hair

Profile: Do you have to wash your hair every day?
Is your skin oily, or was it oily during your teens?
Does your hair look stringy and lank soon
after washing?

Explanation: Oily hair very simply means that the glands are pumping too much oil, causing your hair to have its own oil crisis. It is one of the most common complaints we hear, and it is often associated with fine, thin hair. With this type of hair, there is less hair to absorb the oil, so it shows more quickly.

Oily Hair Care Program

Shampoo: Shampoo your hair every day, if necessary. If you have fairly thick hair, use a shampoo formulated for oily hair. Every 7-10 shampoos switch to a protein shampoo for the next 3-4 washings. If you have fine hair, an oily shampoo is too harsh, so stick with a protein shampoo.

Conditioners: In general, conditioners are not recommended—you have enough oil. But if you find your hair ends becoming dry with constant shampooing, use a conditioner just at the tips of your hair. Never touch the scalp with a conditioner.

Cut and Style: Oily hair is easier to handle when worn short to medium length. Also, keep extremely oily hair off the face, especially if you have skin problems.

More tips: Since heat stimulates your oil glands, limit your use of hot rollers and use a blow dryer on *cool* or *warm* setting.

Dry Hair

Profile: Does your hair have a great deal of static electricity?

Is your scalp often tight?

Does your hair seem dull?

Explanation: Dry hair can be caused by chemicals, overexposure to the sun, or improper use of hair appliances. When your hair is dry, it lacks moisture: either your glands are not producing enough oil or you are somehow stripping the hair of moisture.

Dry Hair Care Program

Shampoo: Use a protein-base shampoo and/or a shampoo formulated for dry hair.

Conditioners: Use an instant conditioner every time you shampoo, making sure you run it through the ends. Use the Blackstrap Molasses-Climatress treatment (see page 83) at least once a month. If your hair is dry due to chemicals, use the treatment once a week until you notice a substantial improvement.

Cut and style: If your hair is quite dry and brittle, then go to a medium or short length, which requires a minimum amount of exposure to the blow dryer. Ideally, you should select a wash-and-wear style. Trim your ends often.

More tips: Brush your hair daily to distribute oil, but do it gently or you will break your hair ends. Massage is essential to stimulate oil glands.

In the summer, protect your hair from the sun by using hairdressing cream. In the winter, if you're bothered with static electricity or a slight frizziness, rub the palms of your hands together so there is some oil, and smooth down your hair. It's a temporary measure, but it works!

Fine, Limp Hair

Profile: Have you been told you have baby's hair?

Does your hair lack body?

Does it seem to fall one-half hour after you leave the house?

Explanation: Fine hair can often be as smooth as silk and have a wonderful sheen, but unfortunately the pluses stop there. This kind of hair has a tendency to get oily, not hold a curl, and look deflated.

Fine, Limp Hair Care Program

Shampoo: Use a mild, protein-base shampoo. Do not use a shampoo for oily hair, even if that is a problem. Your hair is much too fragile for that formula.

Conditioner: If your hair ends are dry, use a conditioner as often as needed. Use a deep-conditioner every 4-6 weeks for extra body. But don't use cream rinses or shampoos combined with conditioners in one bottle—they will make your hair much too soft.

Cut and style: You will be much happier if you realize that there are certain things you can't do without becoming a slave to this hair type. You can't make it stay curly (without a permanent) and you can't wear it too long because the weight of the hair will make it even more limp. However, you can have a beautiful blunt cut, say chin length, and perhaps go into a shorter, layered style for summer. Either of these styles will make you look as if you have more plentiful, fuller hair.

More tips: When blow-drying your hair, get it about 60% dry, then spray on a small amount of setting lotion and finish drying. Used in this fashion, the lotion gives body more effectively, and your hair will not feel coated.

Consider a permanent for extra volume. Henna or color will also add body.

Frizzy or Curly, Coarse Hair

Profile: Is your hair stiff and unmanageable?
Do you sometimes have trouble getting a brush through your hair?
Does a change in the weather seem to make your hair more curly or frizzy?

Explanation: This kind of hair is most often inherited, so if you don't like it, blame your parents and grandparents. What makes the frizz or curl is the structure of the hair itself, so there is little you can do to change the situation. With proper care, however, you can better deal with your hair.

Frizzy or Curly, Coarse Hair Program

Shampoo: Use a protein- or oil-base shampoo.

Conditioner: You need conditioners more than anybody else. After every shampoo use a cream rinse and detangler, which will make your hair softer and more manageable. Use a deep-penetrating conditioner every 1-2 weeks. If your hair ends feel especially dry, use a hairdressing cream.

Cut and style: If you want to go "natural," a short layered cut with a cap of curls is becoming. But if you are more interested in reducing frizz and curl, you will need the weight of a longer style.

More tips: Do not rub your hair vigorously with a towel. The friction will tangle the hair and create more frizz.

Hair Straightening

Hair straightening is a very bad idea; we do not do it in our salons. It's potentially the most damaging thing you can do to your hair. Chemically, straightening lotion is very close in strength to a depilatory, and if left on too long it can dissolve your hair much as a depilatory does. We've seen a number of home-straightening jobs result in bald spots, scalp breakout, and extreme loss of hair. Rather than hair straightening, don't overlook another solution—the right haircut. Try a combination cut—blunt cut in back, layered in front. The cut and the length of this style, worn collarbone length, will naturally "relax" your curl. If you have fine, frizzy hair, then a curly perm will turn most of that frizz into curl. No, it won't be straight hair, but curls may make you happier than frizz.

Chemically Treated Hair

Using chemicals does not necessarily mean that you will have dull or broken hair. But it does mean that you must develop a regular schedule of hair care and stick to it. If you allow chemicals to abuse it, you will have to work that much harder to make your hair look good again.

Chemically Treated Hair Program

Shampoo: If your hair is color-treated, use a shampoo specially formulated for that hair type. If you have had a permanent, use a protein-base shampoo.

Conditioner: Treated hair needs superconditioning. Use an instant conditioner every time you shampoo. For the first month after you put chemicals on your hair, use a deep-penetrating conditioner at least once a week, then taper off to every three weeks or so if your hair is in good shape.

More tips: Don't overexpose your hair to sun or salt water. Limit your use of heat appliances. Handle your hair very gently.

Thin or Thinning Hair

If your hair is thin and has been that way since you were a child, then it is most likely a hereditary condition. But if you find that your hair is beginning to thin, it may be due to many things, such as pregnancy, extended illness, or the birth-control pill. (For further remarks about hair loss, see Chapter 6.) Your hair is extremely fragile, so handle it gently.

Thin Hair Program

Shampoo: Hair should be washed as often as necessary with a very mild shampoo. Never use a detergent shampoo. Also, try not to abuse your hair while washing.

Conditioner: After every shampoo use a conditioner, but use only ¼-½ of the prescribed amount.

Cut and style: Don't wear your hair too long; the heaviness might cause you to lose even more. Strive for a style that is soft and natural, preferably "wash and wear." If you have thinning spots or a receding hairline, don't wrap the hair in an unnatural direction as a cover-up. And don't wear your hair pulled back tightly. (For more information on receding hairlines, see Chapter 2.)

More tips: Don't use a hot blow dryer or hot rollers on your hair. If you must use a dryer, make sure the setting is *cool* or *medium*. Don't brush your hair; use a wide-tooth comb with rounded tip. Increase your circulation with a daily massage.

Combination Hair: Oily Scalp, Dry Ends

Although you may think you are suffering from the worst combination, this is not really a difficult problem to correct. Actually, it is an oily hair condition that is often associated with long hair. Your scalp is producing generous amounts of oil, but the oil is not getting down the hair shafts. You might even be aggravating the condition by using a shampoo for oily hair; it only robs your hair ends of any oil that might be there. Forget the scalp and concentrate on moisturizing the ends.

Combination Hair Program

Brush your hair frequently, so that the oil goes to the hair ends.

A daily massage is a must.

Wash your hair only with a protein shampoo.

Every time you shampoo, use an instant conditioner on the hair ends only. Use a deep-conditioner on the ends anywhere from once a week to once a month, depending on how dry they are.

Limit the use of heat appliances. If you must use hot rollers, always use endpapers.

Trim your hair ends frequently. They are especially prone to damage and split ends when dry.

Dandruff

Dandruff, an annoying problem, can occur with an oily or a dry scalp. Either way, it means that the cells of the scalp are reproducing too rapidly, and as they become too numerous, they fall out as flakes. There probably is no real cure for dandruff. But if you follow a close regimen, you can control dandruff, and at certain times, such as the summer, it may disappear altogether. If it is very stubborn, see a dermatologist.

Dandruff Care Program

Use a shampoo especially formulated for dandruff, such as Selsun Blue, Sebulex, or Head and Shoulders. These shampoos all contain various "anti-dandruff" ingredients, so switch around until you find one that is best for you.

Even after your dandruff is under control, use a dandruff shampoo once every 4 washings.

Once a week, apply Sea Breeze antiseptic to the scalp, leave on for 10-15 minutes, and rinse out. This will remove any loose, dead cells.

Split Ends

In this condition, hairs have split into two or three sections. Consequently, the ends look frizzy and dry. Split ends most often come from harsh treatment of the hair—chemical abuse, overexposure to the sun, or even hard bristle hairbrushes. Split ends are also a common problem among women who wear their hair very long. On hair that is twenty inches long, the ends would be anywhere from two to three years old. No wonder they are dry!

How to Help Split Ends

The most effective measure for split ends is to trim them. Hair will not grow beyond a split end, so don't think you're sacrificing length. And a bad split will only move up the hair shaft, continuing to ruin your hair's appearance.

Use a protein-base shampoo.

Condition those ends like mad. Use an instant conditioner or cream rinse every time you shampoo, and use a deep-penetrating conditioner on the ends at least once a week.

Use a hairdressing cream.

Dull Hair

There are many reasons why your hair may be dull and appear lackluster. If you have a history of too much coloring, too-frequent permanents, or excessive use of hot rollers, don't expect your hair to shine. Also, if you are not rinsing enough after a shampoo, or if you have used regular soap to wash your hair, you are going to have lifeless hair.

"Make Your Hair Shine" Program

Stop excessive use of harsh chemicals, and give your hair a rest.

Condition your hair every time you shampoo, and once a month use a deep-penetrating conditioner. Finish each shampoo with a cool-water rinse.

If you have not used any chemicals on your hair, then you might try a highlighting shampoo in a color near your own shade to add temporary sparkle and shine. This is not a permanent solution to a dull-hair problem.

Make sure there is oil in your diet. Eat avocados, nuts, and a daily salad with oil and vinegar dressing.

Proper Use of Styling Equipment

The next step in attaining *the look* is the proper use of styling equipment. Styling equipment is much more important now than it was ten years ago, when rollers and clips were used for any hairstyle. Then, the idea was to tease and force the hair into a style and hold it that way for a week with hair spray.

Today's approach is more natural. We no longer think in terms of creating a hairstyle with equipment. Instead, a precision cut creates the style by following the natural texture of the hair. The styling tool merely dries the cut into the shape.

Today's hair appliances, such as blow dryers, curling irons, and heat lamps, are no more difficult to use than rollers and clips. Like anything else, it is a matter of getting the hang of it; after that, it becomes second nature. Using appliances will be much easier if you keep in mind that you are trying to achieve a natural shape, not a "set" look.

Blow Dryer

What a blow dryer is good for: Drying hair, making it smooth, curling it, giving it a lift, achieving a contemporary look.

Brands we like: Clairol's Son-of-a-Gun, Hot Stuff, Dry Guy.

When we told our students that we would teach them to blow-dry their hair, a general groan went up. Most of them complained that blow drying was too difficult to master, or that it dried out their hair, or that they needed a third hand to hold blower, brush, *and* hair. As a consequence, we developed several new techniques that make blow-drying hair easier.

Because holding a brush seemed to be a stumbing block, we devised a way to do shorter hair just with the fingers. For longer hair, we found a way to use the brush only at the end of the blowing job. We will also show you other little tricks for blow drying, such as using the palm of your hand to help beat the frizzies.

The secret to an expert-looking blow-dry is to dry the hair

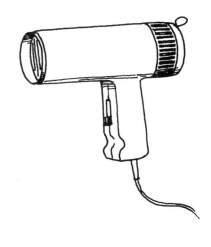

only 95%. A common mistake is to overdry the hair; then you end up with hair that is unmanageable and strawlike.

A good blow dryer can be anywhere from 800 to 1,200 watts, just as long as there is enough power to dry your hair. Lower wattage than this means that you will have to leave the blower on your hair too long. If the wattage is too high, you will be applying unnecessary heat to your hair. If you have fine, thin hair, stay in the lower part of the watt range.

Many blowers on the market are sold with attachments, such as styling brushes and combs. For people with very curly or wiry hair, use the wide-tooth comb attachment as a detangler and the brush for styling. Do not pull the brush through wet hair. If your dryer doesn't come with attachments, we recommend a good styling brush, such as a Denman. This brush features elastic bristles in a molded rubber base. It is flexible enough to move with your hair, and the lack of hard bristles means less chance of hair damage. Here's what kind to get for your particular hair type:

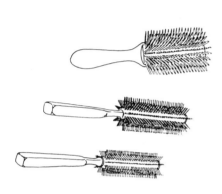

For thick, longish hair: large flat brush (nine-row)

For fine, thin hair: round, small brush

For curly or wavy hair: large round brush

Preliminaries to Blow-Drying

1. Shampoo hair, rinse well, and condition. Towel-dry hair gently so that it is not dripping wet.

2. Using a wide-tooth comb, start at the nape of the neck and comb hair smoothly so that it has no tangles and snarls.

Blow-drying One-Length Hair Turned Under (Chin Length to Collarbone)

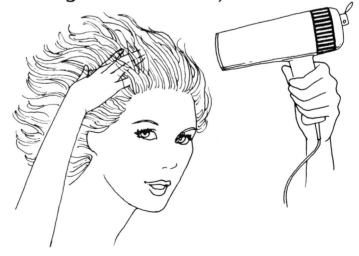

1. Turn the blower on a *hot* setting (*warm* if your hair is fine or processed) and circulate the air throughout the hair. Keep blower moving 8-10 inches away.

2. Run fingers through your hair as you dry and stop blower when hair is about 75% dry.

3. Section the back of the head in half from crown to nape of neck.

4. Divide a 1½- to 2-inch section of hair at the bottom and clip aside the rest. Place the brush in the hair by grasping the end of the hair and rolling the brush under to the scalp, just as if you were placing a curler in the hair. Make sure the brush is secure, but not so tight that it pulls the scalp.

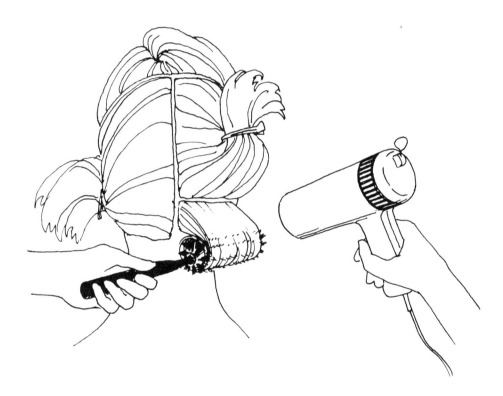

5. Start blow dryer again and aim it on the top of the brush, moving blower back and forth. For those who want more body, aim the blower underneath the brush so that you achieve more fullness.

6. Go to the other side of the back. Take the same-size section and repeat the process.

7. Moving up toward the crown, unclip the next 1½- to 2-inch section of hair. Repeat the process, moving from side to side, until you have finished the entire back.

8. Now move on to the sides, clipping top hair out of the way. Starting once again at the bottom, take a 1½-inch section of hair, roll in brush, and blow from the top. Continue all the way up to the part. Finish one side, then go to the other.

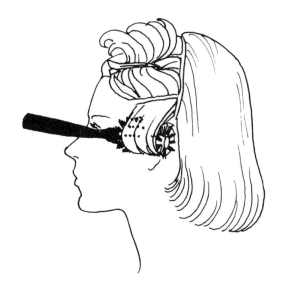

(*Note:* If you have particularly thick hair, you might have to divide the sides into two sections just as you did in the back.)

9. For a different front look, see the special effects section.

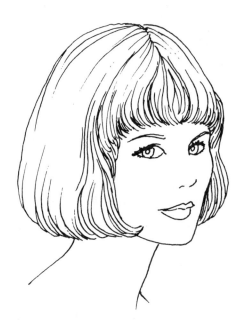

Blow-drying Layered Hair (Straight)

Beginning at the sides, lift each layer with your fingers by starting at scalp and moving to the ends. As you lift each layer and "comb through" with your fingers, follow with the blow dryer. After sides are dry, repeat "lifting" technique in back and then top. This method gives you a soft, natural look and also prevents you from overdrying or damaging your hair because your fingers act as a heat gauge.

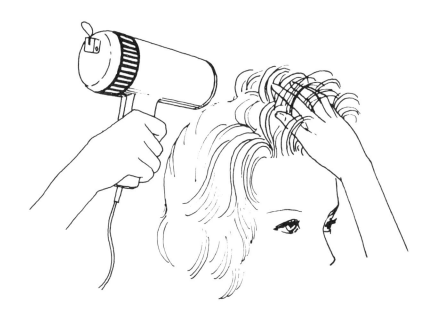

Blow-drying Layered Hair (Curly)

Use the same "lifting" method as described for straight hair until hair is about 50% dry. Then go back over each section and curl hair into the shape you desire with a brush and blower.

Blow-drying Curly Hair
(Smooth Look; Medium Length to Long)

To make curly hair smooth with a blow dryer, always work with wet hair and grasp hair firmly with the brush.

1. Section in half the back of the head from crown to nape of neck.

2. Divide a 1½- to 2-inch section of hair at the bottom. Clip aside the rest.

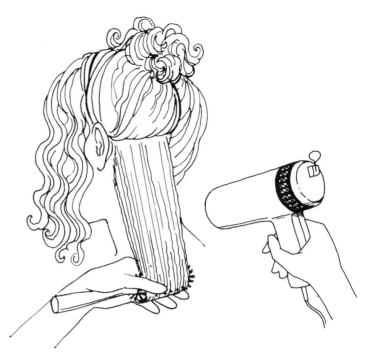

3. Roll brush very firmly into hair. Start blower moving back and forth along the brush on top and underneath.

4. Go to the other side of the back. Take the same-size section and repeat the process.

5. Unclip the next 1½- to 2-inch section of hair. Repeat the process, moving from side to side until you have finished the back.

6. Do each side, starting at the bottom and moving up to the part.

7. Tip for front: If you want to frame your face with hair that is especially smooth, blow-dry hair in the opposite direction, then brush back into place.

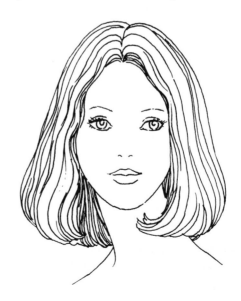

Frizzies or Small Hairs That Won't Cooperate

Sometimes a few small hairs stick up in an otherwise perfect blow-dry. The temptation is to cut them, but that will only make the situation worse. Instead, rub the palms of your hands together so that you get some oil. Turn on the blower, hold from above, and aim hot air at the stubborn ends as you simultaneously stroke them down with your palm. The combination of the heat and oil will coax these little hairs into place.

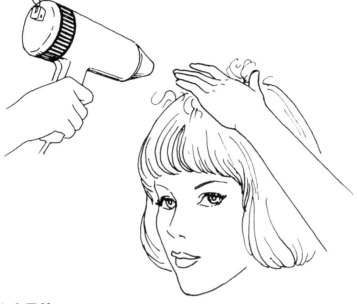

Special Effects

Straight Bangs. Blow bangs back until they are 75% dry. Then bring them forward, holding brush down firmly on bangs. Direct blower from the top. When you have finished, smooth bangs down with the palm of your hand.

Full Bouncy Bangs. Blow bangs back until they are 75% dry. Then bring them forward and roll brush into them from underneath. Move blower back and forth. Remove brush gently.

Side Bangs. Blow bangs back until they are 75% dry, then brush to the side and blend in with side hairs.

Face Framing. You can certainly style hair around your face with a brush, but for a natural look and a method that is fast and easy, try this. Blow-dry all your hair except a 1-inch strip of hair that frames your face from ear to ear. Starting at your part, take a small section of hair and twist it from the root down to the end, like a long piece of spaghetti. Run the blower up and down the length of twisted hair. Then release gently. What you will get is more lift and bounce to your hair and a slightly waved effect. This trick works for a variety of hair types and is especially suitable for slightly wavy, chin-length hair.

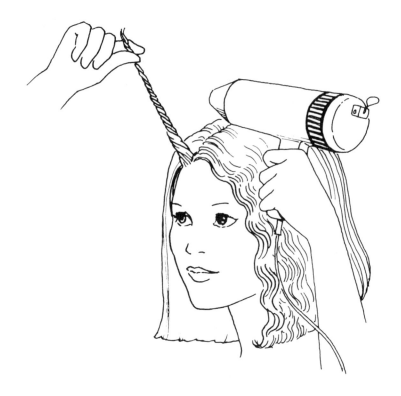

If You're Still Having Problems Blow-Drying

Check your haircut. We promise you that at least 50% of your blow-drying problems will disappear with the right cut. In fact, if you have a good haircut, you won't even have to do a perfect blow-dry job. The hair will fall into place naturally.

Make sure that you have rinsed out all the shampoo from your hair.

Never take too much hair on the brush. Roll as if you were using a roller.

Once you have rolled the brush into your hair, make sure it stays there. It's the blower that moves, not the brush.

Hot Rollers

What they are good for: Add extra body and bounce, set holds better, creates curls in short order.
Brands we like: Clairol.

Hot rollers came out about ten years ago and were highly popular. Originally they were meant to perk up a hairsetting, but most women used them to create a set. We really do not like to see our clients use hot rollers more than three times a week. They can dry out your hair, and if your scalp is oily, constant use of hot rollers will make it even oilier because the heat stimulates the oil glands.

Make sure that you are using the hot-roller kit that is right for your hair. If your hair is hard to curl, then use the dry model of hot rollers. But if you have fine or chemically processed hair, use a steam-conditioner model. Here are some rules that we think are essential to maintaining hair health when using hot rollers.

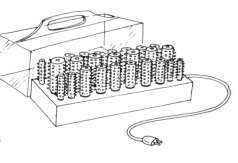

Hot-Roller Commandments

1. Never use hot rollers on wet hair. Blow-dry your hair first.

2. After you have rolled them into your hair, stay still. This is not the time to start doing your exercises. You will yank hair out at the roots.

3. If you have fine or straight hair, spray on a small amount of setting lotion before putting in the rollers.

4. Use endpapers. This will protect your ends from drying out, and loose ends won't stick up in the final set.

5. If your hair is fine or colored, take out the first curler as you put in the last one. Either of these hair types takes a set quickly.

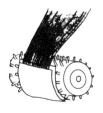

6. For medium or thick hair, leave rollers in for 10-15 minutes or until they are cool. If it seems done to you, take a spot check in the front and back.

7. Most kits come with three roller sizes: large rollers for looser waves, medium rollers for firmer waves, and small rollers for curls and ringlets.

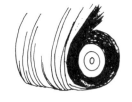

8. Remove rollers gently—don't tangle and snarl the hair. Work from bottom up.

9. Make sure hair is cool before brushing out the set. If hair is thick, bend over and brush out the set. If hair is fine, you may want just to run a comb through the set.

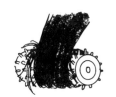

10. Condition your hair often, and cut it regularly. Every 6 weeks is not too often to trim the ends that will be taking the most abuse.

A Word About Rollers

In our opinion, regular rollers are a waste of time and effort. The look you want to achieve is soft and casual, and regular rollers put an artificial structure into the hair. Rollers are also great time-consumers. One of the advantages of today's hair appliances is that they produce the look you want quicker and better.

If you must use something other than a styling appliance, try pin curls as a means of achieving today's soft look. Pin curls

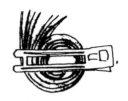

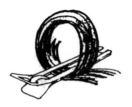

are especially good for heavy or fine straight hair, although you can use them with just about every hair type. Make sure that the clips you use are fresh with no broken tips that can pull at your hair.

There are two basic methods of doing pin curls:

Stand Up: Pull the strand of hair to a 45-degree angle from the scalp. Roll toward head so that curl stands up. This curl should be used in the areas where you want height.

Flat: Roll pin curl toward head and secure with clip. For loose waves, use large strands of hair; for tighter waves or curls, take smaller sections of hair.

Heat Lamps

The newest addition to styling appliances, heat lamps are used to maintain the natural movement of the hair. They give wavy or curly hair a very loose, natural look. People who use heat lamps generally have the least amount of hair breakage.

Heat lamps are actually infrared lamps. You can buy the bulb alone, which screws into a regular light fixture, or you can buy a clip-on light socket at your hardware store or an entire stand at a beauty supply house. We recommend using two bulbs, positioned at either side of your head.

How to Use

1. After shampooing and conditioning, blot excess water with a towel. Comb hair into place, exactly as you want it to look.

2. Place yourself between the two lamps or bulbs, so that you're about 18 inches from either lamp.

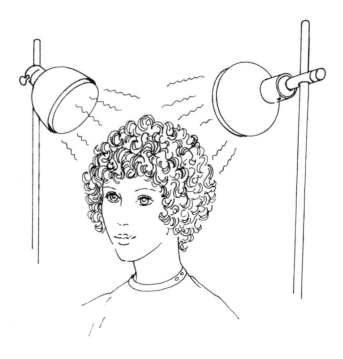

3. As the hair begins to dry, gently fluff up the hair with the tips of your fingers. This will help shape your hair.

4. Stay under lamp 10-20 minutes.

5. Comb through hair.

Curling Irons

After an absence on the styling scene, curling irons are back and have started to regain popularity. Although curling irons can be used to do a whole head, we would rather you use them as an extra tool for styling—to pick up a deflated style or add a few curls or tendrils to a blow-dry style. The advantage to using curling irons is that you can put curls exactly where you want them. They are also great for adding bounce to bangs. Women who color their hair, especially blondes, should be careful using a curling iron. The same applies to women with very fine, thin hair.

Look for curling irons that use steam and have a Teflon wand so that no metal touches the hair. Make sure the unit has a built-in thermostat to keep temperature constant, such as Clairol's Crazy Curl.

How to Use

Comb out a dry strand of hair and secure it under the clip on the curling iron. Make sure that all your ends are under the clip, otherwise they will stick out after you are finished. Roll the curl toward the scalp, stopping ½ inch short. Press the steam button and hold the iron in place for 8-10 seconds. Unwind the iron in one turn and release the curl. Then go on to the next strand and repeat the procedure. For tighter curls, use narrower strands of hair. Unplug the curling iron as soon as you have finished with it. Then gently comb hair into place or just leave it tousled.

4.

How to Give Yourself a Permanent

When they were introduced over twenty-five years ago, permanent waves entailed long complicated processes with often unpredictable results. But today's perms are safe, easy, and they are seeming miracle workers, since they change the hair's very texture. Fine hair can look thicker, limp hair will have more body. If a perm is done correctly, hair will continue to look healthy and will hold its line much better. But if a permanent is done the wrong way, you're in for trouble. Poor permanents will dull and dry the hair to the point where it becomes so brittle that it breaks off.

Caution where permanents are concerned cannot be overemphasized. If you cut your bangs too short, that's too bad, but in only a short time they will grow back to the length you want. However, if you goof while using chemicals, it can be quite a while before your hair is back to normal!

We don't mean to scare you—a perm can certainly be done at home successfully. We just want to impress you with the fact that a permanent must be taken seriously because of its chemical properties.

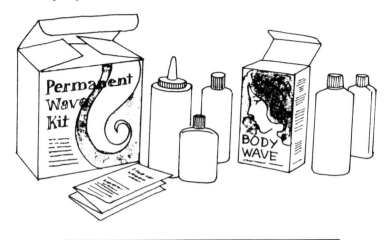

Considering a Permanent?

Do you really need a perm? Check these guidelines before you decide.

The answer is yes, if . . .

- You want to change your look

- Give limp hair body

- Make thin hair look thicker

- Give straight hair waves or curls

- Bend fine frizzies into curls

The answer is no, if . . .

- Your hair is excessively dry or broken

- Your hair is bleached

- You have henna on your hair

- You're under sixteen

- What you really need is a good haircut

What actually happens in a permanent is quite simple. Hair is wound on special rollers (called *rods*), and a waving solution is applied to the hair. After an indicated length of time, the solution is rinsed out, and a neutralizing solution is applied to the hair. The neutralizer does just what its name implies—stops the curling action and keeps hair in its new curly shape.

Types of Permanent Waves

Selecting the right type of permanent is important if you are to get exactly what you are looking for. Basically there are two types of permanents: a body wave, which gives bulk to the hair; and a permanent wave, which gives curl or waves to the hair.

Body waves are used most often at our salons, and we recommend them for home use. They give bulk to fine, thin hair. However, if you want a style with a definite curl, then you must select a permanent wave. There are three types of permanent-wave kits: normal to wavy (for regular hair), gentle (for fine, processed, or gray hair), hard-to-wave (for coarse hair).

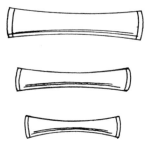

The size of the rods is an important determinant in giving you the style you want. Small rods produce tight curls, while large rods produce loose waves.

Get Ready to Perm

Before we give the go-ahead for any of our clients to have a permanent, we carefully check the hair's condition. If we find that it is slightly dry or has some broken and split ends, we insist on a few deep conditionings before perming, about a week apart, for two weeks or until the hair is no longer dry. If hair is really badly broken, then we forget about the permanent, cut off all the broken ends, and wait until the hair improves. Even if your hair is in good shape, it is important to do a little conditioning before you have a permanent.

One further bit of advice: Don't plan a permanent during your menstrual period or throughout a pregnancy. Because of hormonal changes in your body, a permanent given at these times may not take properly.

Pre-perm Program

Three weeks before your permanent, give yourself weekly deep-penetrating treatments with either Clairol's Condition Beauty Pack Treatment or with our Blackstrap Molasses-Climatress solution as described on page 83.

Don't cut your hair unless it is really out of line and needs three inches or so cut off. In that case, cut off two inches and cut that last inch after the permanent.

Don't color your hair before your permanent. Coloring should be done no sooner than two weeks after a permanent wave, so that your hair has a chance to rest.

Necessary Equipment

1. Complete kit instructions. Just because you have given yourself a perm before, do *not* assume that different brands all work the same way.Make sure you do a test curl. You should know exactly how long it takes to give your hair a permanent wave.

2. A timer. A plastic tail comb. Cotton. Endpapers, if they don't come with the kit.

How to Perm (With Special Salon Tips)

1. Wash your hair with a mild protein shampoo. Lather only once. Towel dry. Condition with Redken's Climatress and rinse out.

2. Block your hair in sections for the rods as shown in the kit's illustration. Section off a 2-inch strip running from the forehead to the crown of the head (1), a strip from the crown to the nape of the neck divided into 2 sections (4 and 7), 2 more strips one on each side (2 and 3), 2 more strips from the crown to the nape of the neck divided into 2 sections (5 and 8, 6 and 9)—9 sections in all.

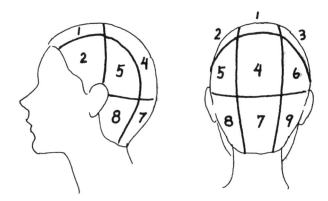

3. Using the rods provided in the kit, set your hair in the desired style.

4. Start rolling rods in front, going toward the back. Use a

tail comb to separate hair, and use only the rollers provided in the kit.

Tips: Hold hair to be rolled straight up and then wrap ends with *wet* endpaper. This is especially important so that hair does not bunch up and create "hooked ends"— the first sign of a home-done job. Don't stretch the hair too tightly on the rods—stop ¼ inch away from the scalp. Too much tension might cause hair breakage, and you might also end up with the frizzies. Try to roll each rod evenly.

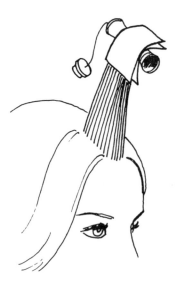

5. After setting, make sure all the rods are in securely enough to hold throughout the entire operaton.

   Tip: Your hair should be dry at this point. If not, take a blower and dry your hair but stop short of total dryness.

6. Wrap cotton all around face and neck to catch any drippings.

7. Starting at the crown, apply the waving lotion to the back area of the hair first and then to the sides and top. It is important to do the back first because this is the hardest area to wave. Cover each curl evenly.

   Tip: Add Redken's P.P.T. "S-77" to the waving lotion. Shake well. We recommend this highly because it acts as a conditioner and reduces some of the waving lotion's alkalinity.

8. Leave the waving lotion on for the length of time indicated in the directions.

   Tip: During this time, do not move around too much or

you will disturb the rods. Also, make sure that you are not in a breeze or even in a hot kitchen—temperature affects the waving lotion. In the salon we place a towel over the client's head. You should do the same at home.

9. When the prescribed time is up, quickly take out a curl at the back behind the ear. Hold curl at the root and pull. If it is shaped like a big S—then you're done. If not, rewrap on rod and leave in for 3 minutes. Test again.

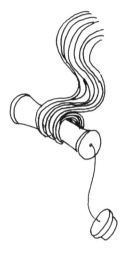

10. When your curl has taken, thoroughly rinse hair—while still in rods—with lukewarm water. Here's where a spray attachment comes in handy. Blot excess water with a towel and change cotton.

11. Apply neutralizer to lock in the curl. Use exactly as the waving lotion, saturating each rod evenly. Keep on for length of time stated in instructions.

12. Rinse out neutralizer thoroughly with lukewarm water.

13. Take out the rods very gently, and using a large plastic comb, sweep all the hair back from the face.

    Tip: Apply Redken's Climatress for 10 minutes and rinse out.

14. Place the hair into shape and dry naturally if it is short; use a blower to dry if it is long.

Tips for Special Hair Types

Fragile or thin hair often takes a permanent quickly. When you do a test curl, you may find that you need to keep the waving solution on only 5-7 minutes.

Hair that is difficult to wave or curl is often thick and coarse. Sometimes the curl will take more quickly in one area than another. If this is the problem, check for the S-shaped curl in the back, on the sides, and on the crown. If you find that your sides and front have taken, but your back has not, then immediately mist water on the areas already "set." This stops the waving lotion while the rest catches up. If there is really quite a difference in the S formations between areas, also apply a waving lotion to the slow-taking area.

What to Do if You Make a Mistake on Your Perm

Underprocessing simply means that you rinsed the waving lotion out too soon. It should not happen if you check for the S-shaped curl. Treat your hair to several deep conditionings and then repeat the permanent waving process. Your hair might take more quickly this time, so test a strand after 5 minutes.

Overprocessing. If you go wrong with a permanent, it is better to take it out too soon than too late. But if you have overprocessed your hair, it will look tightly curled when wet, then frizzy when dry. It will be extremely dull and brittle, and it might even look like steel wool. Here is something you can do, other than buying a wig.

Wait a few days, and during that time use Clairol's Deep-penetrating Condition Beauty Pack Treatment three or four times. Then, on clean, freshly washed hair, apply the wave lotion, mixed with Redken's P.P.T. "S-77." (Don't put in the rods.) With a wide-toothed plastic comb, comb through the hair so that it is saturated right down to the ends. Make sure

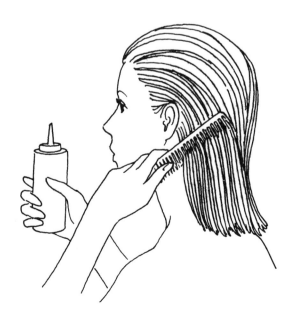

to comb the hair down very flat. After 2-5 minutes (depending on the length of your hair and how overprocessed it is), rinse out. Apply the neutralizer as before, and leave in for 5 minutes. Rinse out. In effect, what you have done is to reverse the permanent process; you should now have body, with a little curl. But recognize that with all these chemicals, the hair has taken a beating, so start immediately on an intensive conditioning program.

Body Perm Without Rods

Occasionally we have a client with fine hair who wants to wear it in a straight style, but she doesn't have enough body to carry it off. A regular body perm might give her too much body and movement. So we give the perm *without* rods, following the same technique we just described for "overprocessed" hair. Since the rods are what give the hair bend, eliminating the rods will add body but will not add curls or waves. This technique is also good for women who need body added to a short, straight style.

Spot Perm

There seems to be some confusion about "spot perm." Professionally, we use the term to mean giving a permanent wave to certain areas of the hair only. For example, a spot perm may wave only 2 inches around the bottom of the hair, or only the hair that frames the face. A spot perm does *not* mean for you to choose at random areas that seem to need a "lift" and then perm just those areas. If you do this, you will end up with hair that puffs up in one place and, by comparison, lies flat in another. If you seem to have an uneven "lift" to your hairstyle, you probably have the wrong cut for your hair, or the wrong style, or both. Most often, we find that women who complain about not having enough "lift" are really wearing their hair too long.

After the Permanent

Just as you followed a pre-permanent conditioner program, you should establish a post-permanent program. You have just put your hair through significant changes, and in return for that new body and bounce, you must give your hair some special attention:

Do

Use only protein- or oil-base shampoos

Use an instant conditioner every time you shampoo

Use a deep-penetrating conditioner such as Blackstrap Molasses-Climatress once a week for a month (See page 83.)

Don't

Overbrush your hair

Apply high heat to your hair (keep blower on warm setting)

Color your hair for at least 2 weeks

The average permanent wave lasts 2-3 months. How long it lasts depends on how often you cut your hair. Before you decide on another permanent, make sure that all of the old wave is out and reevaluate the condition of your hair.

5.

How to Color Your Own Hair

Along with a good cut, the right hair color will make your hair work wonders for your appearance. The right color can take years off your age, flatter your complexion, and dramatize your hairstyle.

Who should color? Just about anyone who wants to. The majority of women who use haircoloring products want to hide gray hair. But there are also plenty of women who wish nature had endowed them with another hair color.

To do a professional-looking job, you must have one goal: natural-looking results. So avoid anything one-color; natural hair has as many as thirty different shadings. If you have never thought about this, study a child's head of hair. You will see many subtle color differences.

You should also stay away from heavy bleaching or anything that produces a tremendous contrast between your original color and your chosen color. These are dated looks; they also necessitate constant touch-ups.

Thanks to major manufacturers who have spent uncountable hours and money on research and development, home hair coloring is better, safer, and more effective than ever. But the market is also flooded with a vast array of products, and it can be confusing to wade through them. This chapter will give you a brief course on the various hair-coloring techniques, so that you can choose the one that best suits your needs. We will also give you special tips on selecting the right color, how to do touch-ups, and what to do if your coloring job is less than perfect.

Chart 4. Hair Coloring Processes

	Natural	Temporary	
Product	Henna	Highlight Shampoo Color rinse	
What it does	Adds color Adds body Adds highlights	Adds highlights Picks up fading color	
Lasts for	2-3 months	1 shampoo	
Lightens	No	No	
Effect on gray	Blends or covers if you have less than 20% gray	Removes yellow from salt-and-pepper hair	
Special remarks	Contains no chemicals; Makes hair shiny; natural shade of henna deposits no color	Very temporary measure	

Coloring Techniques

You may read a great deal about various methods and treatments, but basically color processes can be divided into five categories: natural, temporary, semi-permanent, permanent, and special effects (e.g., hair painting or highlighting). We will discuss each process in detail in this chapter, but for an overall view, see Chart 4.

Semi-Permanent	Permanent	Special Effects
Shampoo-in Creme formula	Shampoo-in Creme formula	Bleach or toner with cap
Enhances natural color Changes "tonal value"	Used to change color of hair— either lighter or darker	Highlights selected strands of hair, not overall color
4-6 shampoos	Until it grows out or is cut out. Touch-up every 3-4 weeks	Until it grows out. Touch-up every 3-6 months.
No	Yes; contains bleach	Yes; contains bleach
Blends in gray Covers if you have 50% or less gray	Covers gray completely	Can highlight with blond
Good way to break into hair coloring since effects are not long lasting	Either single process (one-step application) or double process (lightening, then toning to desired shade)	Excellent for subtle effects

Natural Coloring

Right now, henna is the big natural-coloring product on the market, but it is hardly new. Henna was first used by the ancient Egyptians. Today, in Europe and Israel, henna is used as a shampoo and conditioner because, besides enchancing natural color, it adds tremendous body and sheen to the hair.

What is henna exactly? Henna is an organic vegetable product that coats the hair shaft. Since it does not contain any chemicals, henna will not give you a big change in hair color. But depending on what shade you use, it can deepen your natural color or add color.

Henna is quite frequently used in the coloring work done in our salons. We are enthusiastic about it for home use because it stops coloring after a certain time, so you can't make any serious mistakes. And most important, since henna is natural, you can't damage your hair using it, as you might with a chemical.

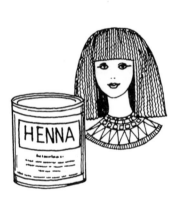

Henna is a white powder that is sold in either packets or cans. Your two best sources are either a health-food store or a beauty-supply house. For best results, henna should be fresh, so do not buy a can that looks as if it has been sitting on a shelf for two years. Two brands that we like and use are Colora and Hopkins.

Henna comes in different shades: black, brown, red, and natural (called *neutral* in some brands). Black henna should be used on very dark heads, while red henna can be used on any shade from dark brown to blonde. Natural henna does not deposit color on the hair, but because it coats the hair shaft, it gives extra body and makes hair look thicker. Also, it will give your hair great shine, as will any henna application. We especially recommend natural henna to people who may not want to change their hair color but do want some extra body.

Chart 5 illustrates the use of henna on different hair colors.

To use henna correctly, read the directions carefully; they differ from one brand to the next. Most instructions tell you to mix water with the henna powder to form a paste, which is then applied to the hair. In our salons we have developed several additional henna mixtures that are easy to apply, and provide extra benefits for the hair.

Chart 5. Henna Results on Your Hair

If Your Natural Hair Color Is	And You Use	You'll Get
Light blonde	Red Natural	Red-blonde highlights Body and shine
Dark blonde	Red Brown Natural	Red highlights Light brown Body and shine
Light brown	Red Brown Natural	Darker brown with red tones Deeper brown Body and shine
Medium brown	Red Brown Black Natural	Red-brown highlights Deeper brown Dark brown Body and shine
Dark brown	Red Brown Black Natural	Red-auburn highlights Deeper brown Black Body and shine
Red	Red Natural	Intensified red Body and shine
Black	Red Brown Black Natural	Red tones Warmer, less dark color Deep black Body and shine
Gray	Natural	Body and shine

Special Henna Formulas

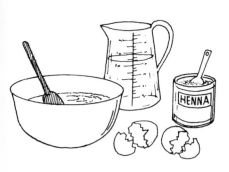

Henna Plus Milk:	3-4 tablespoons milk and 4-6 tablespoons henna. Milk gives extra conditioning to your hair.
Henna Plus Eggs:	1 egg and 4-6 tablespoons henna. A great conditioner, eggs will make your hair feel very soft. This formula is especially recommended for dry hair.
Henna Plus Tea or Coffee (liquid):	3-4 tablespoons tea or coffee and 4-6 tablespoons henna. This makes the henna color darker and richer. It is especially recommended if you are using brown henna on brown hair.

If you use any of these preparations, mix the ingredients to form a paste of medium consistency. It should not drip.

Leave henna on the hair 15-30 minutes for highlights and body and 60 minutes for a definite color change. Henna washes out gradually, but it leaves no "color line." You'll find that henna stays on for 2-3 months.

Temporary Colors

We rarely use temporary colors professionally because they are so short-lived; they wash out with the next shampoo. However, at home you might want to try a temporary color to tone down yellow in salt-and-pepper hair or to pick up a fading color.

Temporary colors fall into two product categories: rinses and highlighting shampoos. The shampoos are made by such companies as Ogilvie and Max Factor, and they are designed to add some highlights. But they contain no peroxide, so there is no lightening effect. For example, if you have medium-brown hair with some red highlights, you can bring them out even more with a red-tone highlight shampoo, such as an auburn-tone.

Color rinses are very often used as a temporary measure to pick up a fading color or to tone down a yellow cast in gray hair. Roux and Clairol both have a wide selection.

Semi-permanent Colors

Semi-permanent colors last through 4-6 shampoos. They will perk up a dull color or enhance your natural shade, but they cannot lighten your hair because they contain no peroxide. Semi-permanents come in two formulas: shampoo and foam. With either formula, follow the manufacturer's instructions.

Because they last through 4-6 shampoos, semi-permanents can be used to change your hair's "tonal" value. For example, if your hair is "warm," in other words, if it has a great deal of red or gold in it, you can use a semi-permanent color in the "ash" family to "cool down" your color. The reverse can also be done, warming up a cool color.

Besides changing the tonal value, semi-permanent colors can also blend or cover up gray, but they do their best job if you are no more than 50% gray. To blend or cover slightly graying hair, choose a semi-permanent color that is the same shade or lighter than your original color. If you are quite gray, and want to cover the gray completely, read the following section on permanent color.

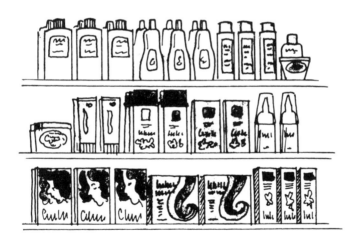

Permanent Color

When you actually change the color of your hair, you use permanent hair color. Unlike the other methods we have discussed, permanent color does penetrate the hair shaft. It can cover gray completely as well as make hair much lighter or darker.

We always explain to clients that permanent color is a commitment. As hair grows in, touch-up work must be done, sometimes as often as every 3-4 weeks.

One-step Permanent Color (also known as Single Process) means that the entire process is done in one step. Most one-step formulas on the market are either shampoo-in or creme. Follow the manufacturer's instructions.

Two-step Permanent Color (also known as Double Process). If your hair is brown and you want to be wheat blonde, two steps are necessary to change your hair color. Step 1 consists of pre-lightening all the color; step 2 consists of toning hair to the desired shade. Famous heads illustrating the two-step process include Catherine Deneuve, Marilyn Monroe, Mae West.

But we are not name-dropping to encourage you to try double-process color. In our opinion, double process is too harsh for the hair. Between bleaching and constant touch-ups, you are just asking for hair breakage. Why pay such a steep price to be blonde?

If your hair is legitimately light brown, you can try using one of the Miss Clairol light blonde shades, which will lift color up to ten shades. You will then be a blonde without having to use the double-process method. But this technique is not for anyone with dark hair.

One last word: If, after all we've said, you still picture yourself as Jean Harlow, *do not attempt it yourself.* Go to the best colorist at the best hairdressing salon you can find.

Special Effects

If you do not want overall color, there are special effects you can achieve. In all these methods, only a few strands are lightened here and there to produce subtle highlights. Hair comes out sun-kissed, as if by nature, rather than from a coloring bottle. Also, these techniques are subtle enough so that when hair grows out, there is no real line of demarcation—quite an advantage! This eliminates the frequent touch-ups that are necessary with overall permanent color.

The following processes are all related, although they produce different results.

Hair painting refers to lightener applied to the hair with a

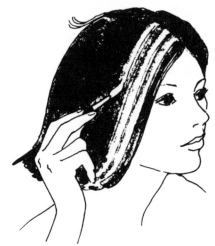

brush. Streaks of color are placed on the outer layers of the hair, following the line of the hair style. Hair painting usually works best on lighter shades. For the most natural results, choose hair only 3-5 shades lighter than your natural color.

Hair highlighting actually blends (or weaves) color throughout different layers of the hair. To execute, strands of hair are pulled through a cap and then lightened. Hair highlighting can be done on any color hair except black. Brown hair might be brought up to show off red highlights, whereas dark blonde hair may be highlighted to pale blonde.

Hair streaking is more dramatic than highlighting because a greater amount of hair is selected for coloring. Streaking is generally done on hair no darker than medium brown; the strands colored are ¼ inch wide or less.

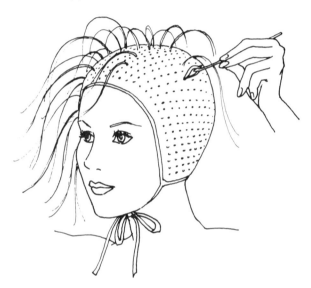

Hair frosting is a similar process to streaking—hair is lightened and then toned. But frosting produces a lighter color because more hair is pulled out through the cap, and the lightener is left on longer.

Hair tipping means lightening only selected ends. Tipping is usually done on short hair.

Note: *Do not* frost, streak, or tip dark hair. You will come out looking like a zebra.

Methods and Products to Achieve Special Effects

Hair painting is done with a brush, but all other special effects are obtained using a cap, which is provided in most home kits. You will be able to recognize these kits quite easily, because they have such names as Frost and Streak, Quiet Touch, or Frost and Tip.

Using aluminum foil is a recent development in producing special effects, and it is the method we use professionally because it gives us better control, allowing us to place the color exactly where we want it. Foil is somewhat tricky to use on your own, however, because you must apply the color to the strands evenly and then wrap them neatly in the foil.

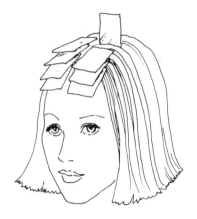

Nevertheless, the cap method will produce perfectly good results if you follow the kit instructions. Some women find it difficult to judge how many strands should be pulled from the cap and exactly where they should be pulled. To take out the guesswork, we have designed some coloring patterns. All you do is trace these patterns on your cap, and you will achieve exactly the coloring effect you want.

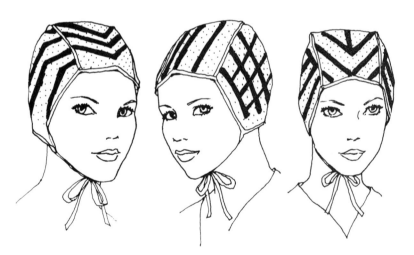

For maximum highlighting.   *Good for layered cuts. Do not use with a center part.*   *Good for blunt cuts.*

Touch-Ups

Highlighting or painting requires the least amount of upkeep. Depending on your base color and how much highlighting you have done, you may be able to go without a touch-up for 3-6 months. With permanent coloring, you may have to have a touch-up every 3-4 weeks because, as your hair grows out, it will show your old color in contrast to the new. This is called showing "roots." The greater the difference between your natural color and your chosen color, the more noticeable the new growth and the more frequent the touch-ups.

When it is time to do a touch-up, do it immediately. All too often we hear women say, "I'll do it next week," or, "In two weeks I'm going to a party, so I'll do it then." Do it *now.* Aside from your hair's poor appearance, if you wait 4-8 weeks, your touch-up may not match the rest of your color. Color "takes" from the heat of the scalp, and if some of your growth is too far from the scalp, it will not take evenly.

To touch-up new growth, follow the manufacturer's instructions carefully. You must be careful not to let the coloring touch hair that has been previously tinted or bleached. If you do overlap, you may notice some spotting or some differentiation of color. Obviously, one-step permanent color is much easier to use at touch-up time than the double process.

Correcting Color Mistakes

Permanent color: If you have made a mistake, do not keep pouring one color after the other on your hair. You will only make matters worse; you could even turn your hair green. Go to a good colorist and let the work be corrected professionally. Besides restoring your appearance, the colorist will show you how and where you went wrong, so you will know for the next time.

Special effects: The usual mistake is that too much hair has been colored. Go to a professional colorist. He will return some of the extra-colored strands back to your former color.

Semi-permanent color: All you need do here to correct your mistake is keep shampooing. The color will wash out more quickly if you shampoo more frequently.

Henna: If you want more color, do the process again, leaving it on for 30 minutes (assuming that you left it on that long to begin with). If your henna came out too red, apply brown henna for 10 minutes and rinse out.

How to Select the Best Color and Product

Choosing a hair color is so involved that it is hard to give general rules. When we choose a hair color for a client in the salon, there are many factors we take into account—condition of hair, base hair color, previous coloring done, reason for coloring, and so forth. But we can give you a few guidelines that should help you to narrow down the field and make a satisfying selection.

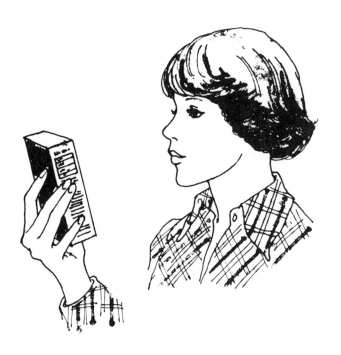

First, decide how much of a change you want. Do you want to cover your gray completely, or do you want highlights? It is a good idea to make small changes at the outset, then work your way into more sophisticated coloring. Second, how much time do you have for touch-ups? You will be doing them yourself, so they will not be costly, but they will be time-consuming. If you are short on time, perhaps you should consider henna. Or if you are medium- to light-haired, one of the techniques described in the Special Effects section, such as highlighting, would be most suitable.

When shopping to select hair coloring, remember that the hair-coloring charts on the packages show shades of color on white hair. Because hair coloring reacts with your own natural color (almost as if you were placing one layer of color on top of another), it will not come out looking exactly like what you see on the chart. For example, if your natural color is medium brown and you want to become a redhead, choose a lighter shade in the red family than the color you actually want.

With all the products on the shelves, do not confuse semi-permanent and permanent products. Semi-permanent colors are complete in themselves; they come in one bottle. Permanent colors, on the other hand, need peroxide and must contain two bottles, the shade and the peroxide. Peroxide may also be called a *booster, developer,* or *activator.*

There are two final considerations when selecting a hair color: age and skin tone. Age is important because as we get older our skin tone becomes more sallow and therefore requires lighter, softer hair coloring to perk it up. In other words, it is unlikely that you will have the same black hair and fair skin at thirty-eight that you had at eighteen. So you might do well to lighten your hair to a warm brown; it will be flattering with your changed skin tone.

When it come to skin tones, remember that in hair coloring "ash" colors refer to cool tones while warm tones are red and gold. If you have a sallow complexion, stay away from ash tones. Fair skin generally needs warm colors. If you are in doubt, try on a few wigs to see how the color looks on you.

Special Tips for Gray Hair

Gray or graying hair is caused by a loss in pigment; that loss makes hair become white or transparent. Sometimes, when hair starts going gray, the rest of the hair looks drab. That is when you can use highlights to brighten up the color.

If gray hair bothers you, by all means cover it up. But very often we advise clients, especially if they have dark hair, to let some of the gray grow in. On some women salt-and-pepper hair looks very smart, and you may like it. But to have gray hair or not is an entirely individual decision, so here are some ideas for shade selection:

If You Are	**Permanent Color** (One-step Process)
Slightly gray	Use the same shade as your original color
Partly gray (35-50%)	1-2 shades lighter than your original color
Mostly gray (50% and over)	5-6 shades lighter than your original color

If your hair is somewhat difficult to cover, try using a creme formula rather than a shampoo-in tint.

Besides permanent color, other color possibilities for gray hair include a semi-permanent tint in a light shade of your natural color to produce a pretty, highlighted effect. In this case the gray will still be there, but it will not be obvious because it will be blended.

Each Time You Use a Color Preparation

Read the label carefully to be sure you are getting what you want in terms of color.

Read directions several times, making sure that you understand the entire process and each individual step. Follow the manufacturer's instructions to the letter; thousands of dollars have been spent to make sure they work.

Have everything you need for the coloring job in front of you. When you are in the middle of mixing is not the time to discover that you are short on peroxide. Also, be sure you have enough time to do the job without interruption.

Do a patch test, even if you have colored your hair before and used the product previously. You may not have had a reaction to a patch test before with a particular product, but products change—and so does your body chemistry. Do a test *each time*.

A strand test is essential in making your home coloring a success. Properly done, it will indicate whether you have chosen the right color and will show you exactly how long the process takes to get to that color. A strand test is especially important on hair that has been given a permanent wave because such hair will be more porous and probably will take color faster.

Color Pointers

After the coloring job, wait at least a day before you judge your new color. Many factors come into play that first twenty-four hours: the natural oils return to the scalp, color oxidizes (reacts with oxygen in the air), and your eyes adjust to the new image. Never study your new color in the bathroom or kitchen or any place where there is fluorescent light.

In our salons the colorist keeps a chart on each client, and we advise you to do the same. Charts note what color preparation was used, how long it stayed on, and the final results. And, of course, the chart includes the date the color was done plus any special notes on hair texture and condition.

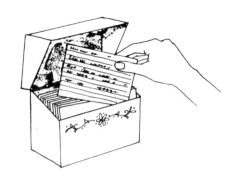

If you plan to color your hair and also have a permanent (which we do not recommend because it can be risky to use two sets of chemicals on the hair), do the permanent first. *Never* do these chemical processes in the same day; it is too much of a strain on the hair. Keep them two weeks apart.

When you change your hair color is the time to reevaluate your makeup as well. This year's red henna does not go with last year's pink lipstick. Another makeup hint: If you have made your hair noticeably lighter, make sure your eyebrows are not too dark. If they are, bleach them out with a preparation specially formulated for this process.

Use a hair conditioner immediately after the coloring job is finished. In fact, we would like to see a crash schedule of conditioning started three weeks before coloring. Give yourself a weekly Blackstrap Molasses-Climatress treatment (see page 83).

As we have stressed throughout this chapter, to be successful at home hair coloring you must understand what you are doing. The color experts at Clairol, with whom we have done a lot of work, have set up a toll-free number where anyone can call with questions and problems on hair coloring. Clairol's hotline number is 800-223-5800, except in New York State, where you call collect to 212-644-2990.

Clairol handles over 100,000 phone calls a year. Because you probably have some of the same questions as those phoned in, we asked Clairol for a list of the most frequently asked questions—and their answers—and we are happy to reprint them here.

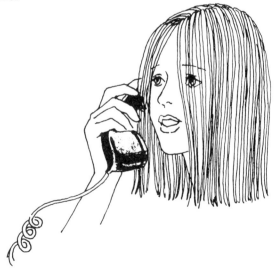

Q. *Is my natural color the color I was when I was young, or is it my color now?*

A. Your natural hair color changes as you change. Therefore, whatever color your natural hair is at the present time, is considered your "natural hair color."

Q. *If I use a shampoo-in tint, will it shampoo out?*

A. No. Shampoo-in hair coloring refers to the method used for coloring the hair. That means you shampoo the color into your hair, wait about twenty minutes (or as long as your strand test dictates), rinse, and you have your new color. The color lasts until the hair grows out.

Q. *I used a hair coloring product several months ago, can I use another color now?*

A. Yes. But take a strand test before applying. Changing colors can be tricky.

Q. *What is peroxide?*

A. Peroxide is the developing lotion that must be mixed with a tint of lightener.

Q. *Will a permanent change my color?*

A. The chemicals in a permanent can lift color.

Q. *Why does my regular tint "take" so dark after I've had a permanent?*

A. Permanent and body-wave solutions tend to make the hair porous. Therefore, less time may be needed for color to "take." Again, that is where your strand test plays a big part.

Q. *Can black people use the same products as whites?*

A. Yes. Choose a product based on your skin color and the texture and condition of your hair.

Q. *Can I use coloring on a human-hair wig?*

A. No. The hair used in human wigs and hairpieces is treated with various chemicals and therefore does not behave like "growing" hair. If you wish to change the color of your wig, it is suggested that you contact your source of purchase for advice on doing so.

Q. *Can my husband use a woman's hair-coloring product?*

A. Yes. And remember, men need hair color just as much as women do—sometimes even more.

Q. *I color my hair. What is a good shampoo for me to use?*

A. For those who use brown or red tints, Clairol Green Colorfast shampoo is the one for you. And, for blondes and gray-haired women, we suggest the Clairol Blue Colorfast shampoo.

6.

Hair Awareness

When an aspiring hairdresser attends beauty school, he first learns facts about the hair itself—what hair is made of, how it grows, what makes it curly or straight. If you are going to do your own hair, we feel that it is important for you to know a little about hair structure and the activity of hair growth. We will talk about these things in this chapter, and will also discuss various factors that contribute to hair loss—what's normal and what's not.

What Is Hair?

Hair is made up of threadlike strands of protein material called *keratin*. Each hair is divided into two sections: the *root*, which is the portion embedded in the skin; and the *shaft*, which is exposed. The shaft is the hair we see as it grows beyond the surface of the scalp.

First, let's examine the hair shaft. (Refer to the diagram as you read along.) The hair shaft grows in three layers, each consisting of cells: the medulla, cortex, and cuticle.

Medulla. This is the innermost layer—a streak running through the center of the hair shaft. It is composed of loosely packed cells with large spaces in between. All the facts about the importance of the medulla are not in yet, but scientists do know that it does not exist in all people.

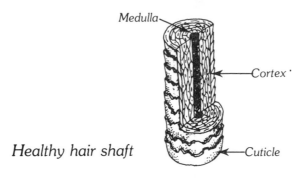

Healthy hair shaft

Cortex. As the middle layer, the cortex consists of long, pointed cells. The cortex is important because it houses the pigment, which gives hair its color.

Cuticle. This is the outer layer of the hair. It is composed of hard, flat cells that overlap, so that they look like fish scales. A flat cuticle makes hair shine.

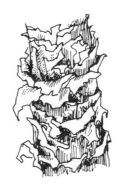

Damaged hair shaft

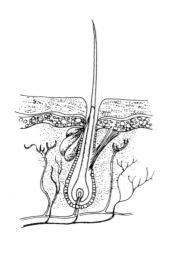

Now let's take a look at the *hair root*. The root is not as simply divided as the shaft, but it is important because it is the very life of the hair. (Again, refer to the diagram.)

Each hair shaft grows out of a root, which rests in a sac called the *follicle*. A hair begins its new life in the follicle, starting out from the very bottom in a place called the *papilla*. The papilla supplies the cells that start the hair growing, and it also draws the necessary elements from the blood to nourish the hair.

What makes hair curly or straight? Now that you understand what hair is, you should be able to comprehend what makes hair straight, curly, or wavy. The differences are created by the shape of the hair shaft and the way each shaft grows in the hair follicle.

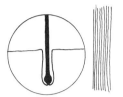 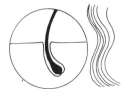 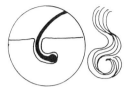

Facts about Hair

Hair fullness depends on the size and shape of the hair shaft and on the number of hairs on the head. As a rule, an individual head of hair runs from 90,000 to 140,000 hairs. Blondes generally have the most hair, averaging 140,000 per head; brunettes average 110,000 hairs per head; and redheads come in lowest, at 90,000 hairs per head. But these are just average figures. It is not unusual to find a blonde with fewer hairs than a brunette.

Hair size: The diameter of a single hair can go from 1/140th of an inch to 1/1500th of an inch, thus making the difference between coarse and fine hair types.

Hair growth: Providing all conditions are right, hair grows about one-half inch per month. There are exceptions, of course. We've seen some people whose hair grows only one-quarter inch a month, while others have hair that can grow as much as three-quarters of an inch per month. Each hair stays on your head anywhere from two to six years and then falls out because it has been pushed out by a new one. Cutting does not make your hair grow faster; it just seems that way because it eliminates split ends.

Hair Loss

A certain amount of hair loss is normal; you probably lose 50-90 hairs when you wash or brush your hair. This means that those hairs were ready to come out anyway. Hair loss is generally lowest during the summer, perhaps because of the better weather. If you are losing more hair than normal, it can be due to a variety of reasons.

Hair might have loosened at the roots from a long illness,

particularly one that involves a high fever, and you may experience some hair loss. Usually, as soon as the body health and nutrition return to normal, so does the hair.

Stress, or tension, can contract muscles and thereby restrict circulation. If you are under a great deal of stress, try massaging your scalp and brushing your hair daily.

You are what you eat, and we have never seen hair that did not benefit from a nutritionally sound diet, including plenty of essential proteins and B vitamins.

Female Hair Loss

Although the effect of the birth-control pill on hair loss is still under investigation, several studies show that there may well be a correlation between the two and just as the body's hormonal balance is disturbed by the pill, so is it affected in menopause. Some women find that they lose more hair at this time.

Most women complain of an accentuated hair loss after pregnancy. This usually means that the body is readjusting; when it returns to normal, so will the hair. Usually, this takes a complete year after the birth.

Male Hair Loss

The most common reason for hair loss among men is male-pattern baldness, or MPB for short. The hair does not actually fall out; it gradually becomes thin and finally disappears. The hairline usually follows a horseshoe pattern on the scalp, but some hair usually remains on the sides and back of the head.

Whether or not your hair loss is due to one of the above-mentioned reasons, you may wish to check with a dermatologist. We would also suggest that you pep up your circulation with scalp massage and use conditioners to protect and strengthen the hair.

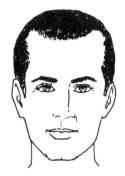 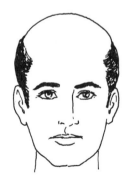

7.

Special Hair, Special Situations

These final pages consist of hair advice and tips based on questions most frequently asked. The categories cover special hair situations that you should be familiar with if you are going to care for your own hair.

Black People's Hair

Although black people's hair is often considered difficult to work with, it really isn't. The important thing is learning how to work with it. Characteristically, black hair is porous and wiry and has a strong wave pattern.

Shampoos and conditioners: Use a mild protein-base shampoo. Do not use combination shampoo conditioners or cream rinses; they will make your hair too soft. However, after every shampoo use an instant conditioner such as Redken's Climatress or Clairol's Instant Conditioner. Use a deep-

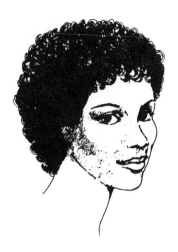

penetrating conditioner once every two weeks for more manageable hair.

Cuts and styles: The newest, hottest style for black men and women is a layered cut with an overall length of 3½ inches. The hair is set on perm rods for a soft, curly look. The large, overblown Afro is out. What's in is a more closely cropped Afro; the hair still looks natural, but neater. Other style possibilities include corn rows and braids.

Children's Hair

Children's hair needs very gentle handling. Because it is still forming, it is much more fragile than an adult's hair. The happier you make a child's hair experience, the better chance you will stand of having a well-groomed teen-ager.

Special Tips for Children's Hair

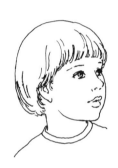

When cutting a child's hair, do it slowly; never yank or pull at the hair. Also, attempt to cut a child's hair only when your patience level is high.

Use a very mild protein shampoo that does not sting the eyes. If it makes the child more secure, take a thick washcloth, fold it over several times, and have the child hold it tightly over his eyes while you shampoo and rinse.

Always use a cream rinse and detangler when you shampoo your child's hair.

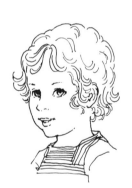

Don't let a child go too long between shampoos if you see the scalp looking oily. Infections start very easily.

If your child goes to summer camp or boarding school, make sure he or she has a simple, manageable haircut and plenty of mild shampoo and cream rinse to take along. Teach your child not to share combs and brushes with other children.

Don't even think of permanents or hair coloring for a child. (We've seen this done to some child models, and it makes us sad.) Children are—and should be—totally natural.

Illness and Your Hair

If illness confines you to bed for a few months, there are special precautions that should be taken to ensure easy hair care and a minimum of damage to your hair.

Switch to a shorter haircut. Or if your hair is long enough, put it into a braid or bun.

Comb through your hair every morning. This is very important to eliminate snarls or tangles.

Circulation is decreased when you lie in bed all day, so give yourself a scalp massage once a day. Using the fat pads of your fingers, gently rub the scalp in a circular motion.

At night, cover your head with a silk scarf. This will decrease the friction that results from rubbing your head on the pillow. Too much friction can loosen hair follicles and cause hair to fall out.

To remove oil, use a dry shampoo until you can get your hair washed.

Travel Tips

You may go off on the vacation of your life and suddenly find that your hair is not having as good a time as you are. Change of schedule and environment can certainly affect your hair, but change of water is often the real villain. Most of us live with hard water, which gives hair body; when we switch to soft water, hair goes limp. If this is really a problem to you, invest in bottled water; that will make hair easier to manage. A change from warm to cold weather produces static electricity, so take along some hairdressing cream to lubricate and protect your hair as well as reduce static electricity.

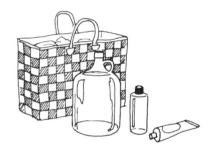

Seasonal Care of Your Hair

Summer

Cover your hair in the sun with a loose, floppy hat, especially if your hair has been chemically treated.

Wash out salt water and chlorine from hair immediately.

Don't get suntan lotion on colored hair; you may end up with a new shade.

While you are sitting in the sun or lolling around the pool, take advantage of the leisure time. Apply a deep-penetrating conditioner, then cover the head.

Try a "wash-and-wear" hairstyle, one that looks good when wet and takes a minimum amount of effort to style.

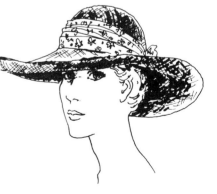

Keep a wide-toothed plastic comb in your beach bag for smoothing out tangles.

Winter

Don't wear tight-fitting wool caps, especially if you have an oily scalp. The heat will make your oil glands more active.

Condition hair regularly. Exposure to dry, cold air can rob your hair of natural oils.

Shampoo hair only once each time you wash.

Beauty Supply Houses

Most of the products we have mentioned in this book can be bought at your local drugstore or supermarket. However, if you want to buy hair products from a beauty supply house, we can give you the name of one we work with in New York—and two others that have been recommended to us.

United Beauty Supply
49 West 36th Street
New York, NY 10036

Paris Beauty Supply
46-32 Santa Monica Blvd.
Los Angeles, CA 90029

Baily Beauty Supply
2243 West Harrison St.
Chicago, IL 60612

Your Hair and the Man in Your Life

Perhaps this is more in the way of personal philosophy than a tip, but we pass it along. All too often, we see women who have been wearing their hair the same way for the last ten years. Their excuse for not updating it is either that "my husband would kill me" or "he likes it this way." Let's face it. Sameness is boring in most areas; why should hairstyles be different? And boredom is a relationship killer. A new hairstyle or a change in color will lift your spirits and affect those around you. So don't be afraid to take the step!

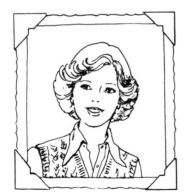

"You Oughta Be in Pictures"

We are ending the book on this note because if you have followed our advice, you *should* have your picture taken. In fact, we took pictures of some of our students at the beginning of the term, and then again at the end. What a wonderful difference.

We hope it is the same for you.